Virtual Clinical Excursions—Pediatrics

for

Wong and Hockenberry:
Wong's Essentials of Pediatric Nursing
6th Edition

prepared by

Marilyn J. Hockenberry, PhD, RN-CS, PNP, FAAN

David Wilson, MS, RNC

Marilyn Winkelstein, PhD, RN

Contributing Editor

Patrick Barrera, BS

Virtual Clinical Excursions Author and Software Design

Jay Shiro Tashiro, PhD, RN
Director of Systems Design
Wolfsong Informatics
Tucson, Arizona

Ellen Sullins, PhD
Director of Research
Wolfsong Informatics
Tucson, Arizona

Gina Long, RN, DNSc
Assistant Professor, Department of Nursing
College of Health Professions
Northern Arizona University
Flagstaff, Arizona

Software Development

Michael Kelly
Developer and Programmer
Michael M. Kelly and Associates
Flagstaff, Arizona

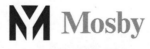

Mosby

An Affiliate of Elsevier Science
St. Louis   London   Philadelphia   Sydney   Toronto

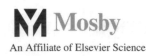
Mosby

An Affiliate of Elsevier Science

11830 Westline Industrial Drive
St. Louis, Missouri 63146

Virtual Clinical Excursions—Pediatrics for Wong and Hockenberry: ISBN 0-323-01946-3
Wong's Essentials of Pediatric Nursing, 6th edition
Copyright © 2003,   Mosby, Inc.   All rights reserved.

Notice

Pharmacology is an ever-changing field. Standard safety precautions must be followed, but as new research
and clinical experience broaden our knowledge, changes in treatment and drug therapy may become necessary or appropriate. Readers are advised to check the most current product information provided by the
manufacturer of each drug to be administered to verify the recommended dose, the method and duration of
administration, and contraindications. It is the responsibility of the licensed prescriber, relying on experience and knowledge of the patient, to determine dosages and the best treatment for each individual patient.
Neither the publisher nor the editor assumes any liability for any injury and/or damage to persons or prop-
erty arising from this publication.

The Publisher

First Edition 2003.

Vice President and Publishing Director, Nursing: Sally Schrefer
Editor, Nursing: Tom Wilhelm
Senior Developmental Editor: Jeff Downing
Project Manager: Gayle May
Designer: Wordbench
Cover Art: Jyotika Schrof

WB/MVB

Printed in the United States of America

Last digit is the print number: 9   8   7   6   5   4   3   2   1

Workbook
prepared by

Marilyn J. Hockenberry, PhD, RN-CS, PNP, FAAN
Director, Center for Clinical Research
Nurse Scientist, Texas Children's Hospital
Director of Nurse Practitioners, Texas Children's Cancer Center
Professor, Department of Pediatrics, Baylor College of Medicine
Houston, Texas

David Wilson, MS, RNC
Staff Nurse, Children's Hospital at Saint Francis
Tulsa, Oklahoma

Marilyn Winkelstein, PhD, RN
Associate Professor
Johns Hopkins University School of Nursing
Staff Educator
Johns Hopkins Hospital Children's Center
Baltimore, Maryland

Contributing Editor

Patrick Barrera, BS
Research Program Coordinator
Clinical Research Center
Texas Children's Hospital
Houston, Texas

Textbook

Donna L. Wong, PhD, RN, PNP, CPN, FAAN
Adjunct Associate Professor, University of Oklahoma College of Medicine—Tulsa
Adjunct Professor, University of Oklahoma College of Nursing
Adjunct Professor/Consultant, Oral Roberts University, Anna Vaughn School of Nursing
Consultant, Children's Hospital at Saint Francis, Tulsa, Oklahoma
Consultant, Texas Children's Hospital, Houston, Texas

Marilyn J. Hockenberry, PhD, RN-CS, PNP, FAAN
Director, Center for Clinical Research
Nurse Scientist, Texas Children's Hospital
Director of Nurse Practitioners, Texas Children's Cancer Center
Professor, Department of Pediatrics, Baylor College of Medicine
Houston, Texas

David Wilson, MS, RNC
Staff Nurse, Children's Hospital at Saint Francis
Tulsa, Oklahoma

Marilyn L. Winkelstein, PhD, RN
Associate Professor
Johns Hopkins University School of Nursing
Staff Educator
Johns Hopkins Hospital Children's Center
Baltimore, Maryland

Patricia Schwartz, PhD, RNC, CPNP
Formerly Director of Nursing Research
Texas Children's Hospital
Houston, Texas

Contents

Getting Started

■ **MINIMUM SYSTEM REQUIREMENTS**

Virtual Clinical Excursions—Pediatrics is a hybrid CD, so it runs on both Macintosh and Windows platforms. To use *Virtual Clinical Excursions—Pediatrics*, you will need one of the following systems:

- **Windows™**

  Windows XP, 2000, 98, 95, NT 4.0
  IBM-compatible computer
  Pentium II processor (or equivalent)
  300 MHz
  96 MB (minimum) of RAM
  800 × 600 screen size
  Thousands of colors
  100 MB hard drive space
  12× CD-ROM drive
  Soundblaster 16 soundcard compatibility
  Stereo speakers or headphones

- **Macintosh®**

  MAC OS 9.04
  Apple Power PC G3
  300 MHz
  96 MB (minimum) of RAM
  800 × 600 screen size
  Thousands of colors
  100 MB hard drive space
  12× CD-ROM drive
  Stereo speakers or headphones

Note: *Virtual Clinical Excursions—Pediatrics* is not designed to function at a 256-color depth. You may need to access the Control Panel on your computer and adjust the Display setting. See specific instructions for this in How to Adjust Your Monitor's Settings on p. 2 of this workbook.

1

■ INSTALLING *VIRTUAL CLINICAL EXCURSIONS—PEDIATRICS*

Virtual Clinical Excursions—Pediatrics is designed to run from a set of files installed on your hard drive and a CD inserted in your CD-ROM drive. Minimal installation is required.

- **Windows™**

    1. Start Microsoft Windows and insert *Virtual Clinical Excursions—Pediatrics* **Disk 1 (Installation)** in the CD-ROM drive.
    2. Click the **Start** icon on the taskbar and select the **Run** option.
    3. Type d:\setup.exe (where "d:\" is your CD-ROM drive) and press **OK**.
    4. Follow the on-screen instructions for installation.
    5. Remove *Virtual Clinical Excursions—Pediatrics* **Disk 1 (Installation)** from your CD-ROM drive.
    6. Restart your computer.

- **Macintosh®**

    1. Insert *Virtual Clinical Excursions—Pediatrics* **Disk 1 (Installation)** in the CD-ROM drive. The disk icon will appear on your desktop.
    2. Double-click on the disk icon.
    3. Double-click on the icon **Install Virtual Clinical Excursions**.
    4. Follow the on-screen instructions for installation.
    5. Remove *Virtual Clinical Excursions—Pediatrics* **Disk 1 (Installation)** from your CD-ROM drive.
    6. Restart your computer.

■ HOW TO ADJUST YOUR MONITOR'S SETTINGS (WINDOWS™ ONLY)

- **Windows 95/98/SE/ME/2000**

    1. Click the **Start** button and go to **Settings** on the pop-up menu. Click on **Control Panel**.
    2. When the Control Panel window opens, double-click on the **Display** icon.
    3. This opens the Display Properties window. Click on the **Settings** tab (on the top right). Below the image of the monitor, you will find the settings for color quality and screen resolution. Change this to **High Color (16 bit)** by selecting it from the drop down menu. On the right is the Desktop area. Click and hold down on the slider button and move it to 800 by 600 pixels. Now click **OK**.
    4. If Windows™ asks you to confirm the change, click **OK**. Your screen will resize and Windows™ may again ask you whether you want to keep these new settings. Click **Yes**.

- **Windows XP**

    1. Click the **Start** button; then click **Control Panel** on the pop-up menu.
    2. Click **Display**. If Display does not appear, click **Switch to Classic View**; then click on **Display** icon.
    3. From the Display Properties dialog box, select the **Settings** tab.
    4. Under Screen Resolution, click and drag the sliding bar to adjust the Desktop size to 800 x 600.
    5. Under Color Quality, choose High or Highest.
    6. Click **Apply**. If you approve of the new settings, click **Yes**.

■ HOW TO USE DISK 2 (PATIENTS' DISK)

- **Windows™**

  When you want to work with any of the five patients in the virtual hospital, follow these steps:

  1. Insert *Virtual Clinical Excursions—Pediatrics* **Disk 2 (Patients' Disk)** into your CD-ROM drive.
  2. Double-click on the icon **Shortcut to VCE Pediatrics**, which can be found on your desktop. This will load and run the program.

- **Macintosh®**

  When you want to work with any of the five patients in the virtual hospital, follow these steps:

  1. Insert *Virtual Clinical Excursions—Pediatrics* **Disk 2 (Patients' Disk)** into your CD-ROM drive.
  2. Double-click on the icon **Shortcut to VCE Pediatrics**, which can be found on your desktop. This will load and run the program.

■ QUALITY OF VISUALS, SPEED, AND COMMON PROBLEMS

Virtual Clinical Excursions—Pediatrics uses the Apple QuickTime media layer system. This includes QuickTime Video and QuickTime VR Video, which allow for high-quality graphics and digital video. The graphics seen in the *Virtual Clinical Excursions—Pediatrics* courseware should be of high quality with good color. If the movies and graphics appear blocky or grainy, check to see whether your video card is set to "thousands of colors."

Note: Virtual Clinical Excursions—Pediatrics is not designed to function at a 256-color depth. To adjust your monitor's settings, see instructions on p. 2.

The system should respond quickly and smoothly. In particular, you should not see any jerky motions or experience unusual delays as you move through the virtual hospital settings, interact with patients, or access information resources. If you notice slow, jerky, or delayed software responses, it may mean that your particular system requires additional RAM, your processor does not meet the basic requirements, or your hard drive is full or too fragmented. If the videos appear banded or subject to "breakup," you may need to find an updated video driver for the computer's video card. Please consult the manufacturer of the video card or computer for additional video drivers for your machine.

If you are experiencing misplacement of text or cursors in the Electronic Patient Record (EPR), it is likely that your computer operating system has enabled font smoothing. Please turn font smoothing off by following these instructions:

- **Windows™**

  From the Control Panel window select **Display** and then select the **Effects** tab. Make sure the "Smooth Edges of Screen Fonts" is unselected.

- **Macintosh®**

  From the desktop, click on the **Apple** icon in the upper left corner. From the drop-down menu, select **Control Panel**; then select **Appearance**. Click on the **Fonts** tab and make sure the selection box next to "Smooth all fonts on screen" is unselected.

Virtual Clinical Excursions—Pediatrics uses the Adobe Acrobat Reader version 5 to display information in certain places in the simulation. If you cannot see any information when accessing the Charts, Medication Administration Record (MAR), or Kardex, it is likely that the Adobe Acrobat Reader was not installed properly when you installed *Virtual Clinical Excursions—Pediatrics*. To remedy this, you can manually install the Acrobat Reader from the *Virtual Clinical Excursions—Pediatrics* **Disk 1 (Installation)**. Double-click the **Adobe Acrobat Reader** installer (ar505enu.exe) on the disk and follow the on-screen instructions. Once the installer has finished installing the Acrobat Reader, restart your computer and then resume your use of *Virtual Clinical Excursions—Pediatrics*.

■ TECHNICAL SUPPORT

Technical support for this product is available at no charge by calling the Technical Support Hotline between 9 a.m. and 5 p.m. (Central Time), Monday through Friday. Inside the United States, call 1-800-692-9010. Outside the United States, call 314-872-8370.

Trademarks: Windows™ is a registered trademark.

A QUICK TOUR

Welcome to *Virtual Clinical Excursions—Pediatrics*, a virtual hospital setting in which you can work with seven patient simulations and also learn to access and evaluate the health information resources that are essential for high-quality patient care. As you use this workbook and software, you will find that the exercises guide you to conduct assessments, to review patient records, and to plan care for your patients.

Canyon View Regional Medical Center, is a multistory teaching hospital with a Well-Child Clinic, Pediatric Floor, Surgery Department, Intensive Care Unit, and a Medical-Surgical Floor with a Telemetry Unit. You will have access to the pediatric patients within the Well-Child Clinic and Pediatric Floor. One patient will also spend time in the Surgery Department, where you can follow him through a perioperative experience.

Although each floor plan in the medical center is different, each is based on a realistic hospital architecture modeled from a composite of several hospital settings. All floors have:

- A Nurses' Station
- Patients, seen either in examination areas or in their inpatient rooms
- Patient records (*Note*: The Well-Child Clinic keeps only one type of patient record—the Chart. However, on the Pediatric Floor and in the Surgery Department, patient records are kept in several formats—the Chart, Kardex plan of care, Medication Administration Record, and Electronic Patient Record.)

■ BEFORE YOU START

When you use *Virtual Clinical Excursions—Pediatrics*, make sure you have your textbook nearby to consult topic areas as needed. Also remember that you must have your Patients' Disk to run the simulations. If you have not already installed your *VCE-Pediatrics* software, do so now by following the steps outlined in **Getting Set Up** at the beginning of this workbook.

■ ENTERING THE HOSPITAL AND SELECTING A CLINICAL ROTATION

To begin your tour of Canyon View Regional Medical Center, insert your *Virtual Clinical Excursions—Pediatrics* Patients' Disk and double-click on the desktop icon **Shortcut to VCE Pediatrics.** Wait for the hospital entrance screen to appear (see below). This is your signal that the program is ready to run. Your first task is to get to the unit where you will be caring for patients and to let someone know when you arrive at the unit. As in any multistory hospital, you will enter the hospital lobby area, take an elevator to your assigned unit, and sign in at the Nurses' Station.

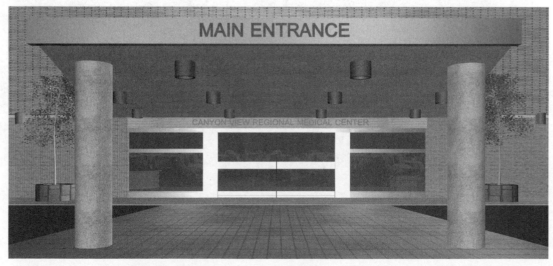

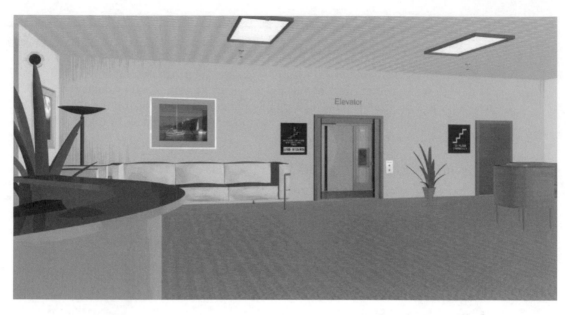

Let's practice getting to your unit in Canyon View Regional Medical Center by following this sequence:

- Click on the hospital entrance door and you will find yourself in the hospital lobby on the first floor (see above).
- Across the lobby, you will see an elevator with a blinking red light. Click on the open doorway and you will be transported into the elevator (see below).
- Now click on the panel on the right side of the doorway. The panel will expand to reveal buttons that allow you to go to the other floors of the hospital.
- Slowly run your cursor across the buttons to familiarize yourself with the different floors and units of the hospital.

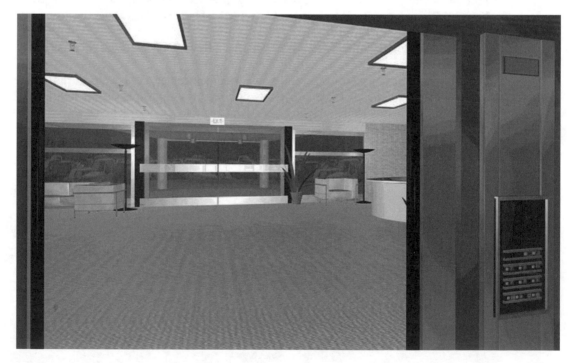

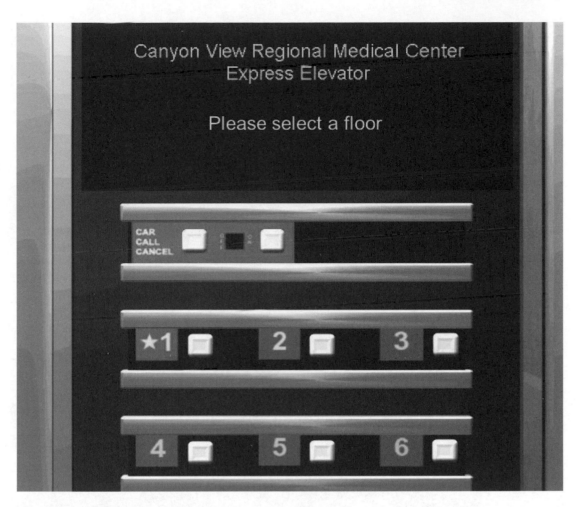

You are currently in a pediatric rotation, so you will not be able to visit the Intensive Care Unit or Medical-Surgical/Telemetry Floor. However, you can work with three children in the Well-Child Clinic, three on the Pediatric Floor, and one who spends time on the Pediatric Floor and in the Surgery Department.

Now, go to Pediatrics and sign in for patient care. To do this:

- Click on the button for the Pediatric Floor (Floor 3).
- The elevator takes you to Floor 3 and opens onto a virtual Pediatric Unit with a Nurses' Station in the center and rooms arranged around the Nurses' Station.
- Click on the **Nurses' Station** and you will be transported inside the station, behind its counter.
- If you click and hold down your mouse button, you can get a 360° view of the Pediatric Floor by dragging your mouse to the left or right. Practice dragging left and right, then up and down, to get a complete view of the Nurses' Station and the Pediatric Floor.
- Take a few minutes to familiarize yourself with the Nurses' Station. First, find the computer with the word **Login** on its screen. This is the Supervisor's Computer, which allows you to select a patient to work with. Now click and drag your mouse to the right or left until you see another computer. This computer allows you to access the **Electronic Patient Records (EPR)** system. Continue browsing around the Nurses' Station until you have found the patient Charts, the Kardex plan of care notebooks, and the Medication Administration Record (MAR).

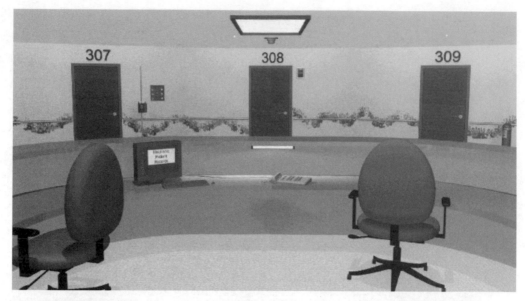

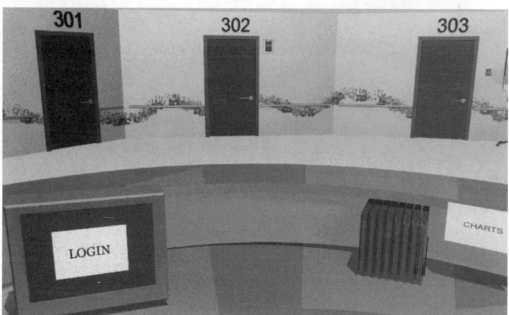

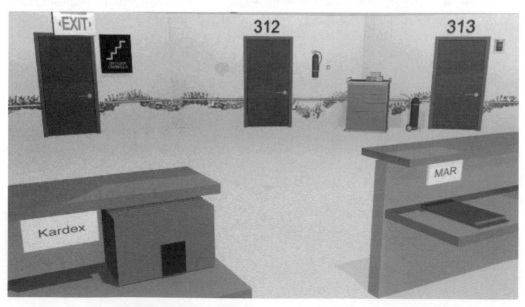

■ WORKING WITH PATIENTS

The Pediatric Floor can be visited from 0700 to 1500, but you can see only one patient at a time and only in specified blocks of time. We call these blocks *periods of care*. In any of the Pediatric Floor scenarios, you can select a patient and a period of care by accessing the Supervisor's (Login) Computer. Double-click on this computer to open the sign-in screen, which contains a box with instructions. Click the **Login** button and you will see a screen that lists the patients on this floor and the periods of care in which you can visit and work with them. Again, only one patient can be selected at a time. When you have completed a period of care with one patient, you can select another period of care for that patient or select another pediatric patient.

Note: During a patient simulation you may receive an on-screen message informing you that the current period of care has ended. If this occurs and you have not yet completed the assigned activities (or if you want to review part of the simulation), simply return to the Supervisor's Computer and sign in again for the same patient and period of care.

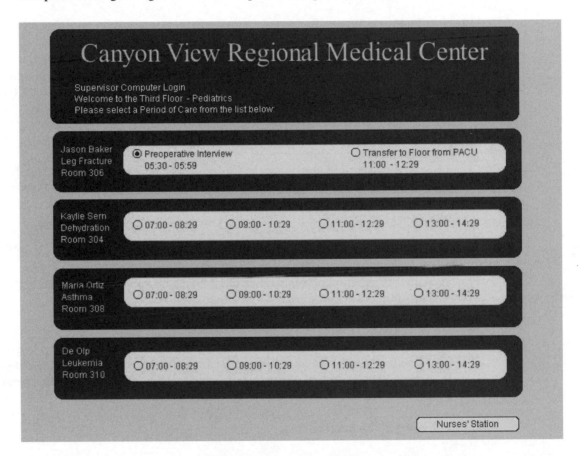

You can choose any of the four patients on this floor (but only one at a time). When you choose a patient, you must also select a period of care. Three of the patients (De Olp, Kaylie Sern, and Maria Ortiz) can be seen during the following four periods of care: 0700–0829, 0900–1029, 1100–1229, and 1300–1429. The fourth patient, Jason Baker, can be seen on the Pediatric Floor from 0500 to 0529 for a preoperative interview. He then goes to the Surgery Department for pre-operative care, surgery, and a period in the PACU (from 0630 to 1029). Jason returns to the Pediatric Floor at 1100, after leaving PACU. You can then see him on the Pediatric Floor from 1100 to 1229. (*Note:* The process of selecting patients is basically the same on all floors of Canyon View Regional Medical Center, although the available periods of care in the Well-Child Clinic and the Surgery Department are different from those on the Pediatric Floor. You will observe this when you visit the other floors. Take a few minutes now to become acquainted with all the patients you will work with.

■ PATIENT LIST

◆ **Floor 2: Well-Child Clinic**

● Paul Parker (Room 202)
Paul is a 24-month-old child visiting for a routine well-child examination. He has a history of ear infections. He is accompanied by his mother.

● Sherrie Bedonie (Room 204)
Sherrie, a 48-month-old child, has come to the clinic for a routine well-child visit. Sherrie's mother is with her throughout the examination.

● Matthew Brown (Room 205)
Matthew is a 10-month-old child. He and his father have come to the clinic for a well-child examination.

◆ **Floor 3: Pediatric Floor**

● Kaylie Sern (Room 304)
Kaylie is a 3-year-old brought to the Emergency Department by her foster mother. She has had a fever and poor appetite for the past 48 hours. Kaylie has a primary diagnosis of dehydration and a secondary diagnosis of acute bilateral otitis media. She was admitted for observation and rehydration.

● Jason Baker (Room 306)
Jason is a 14-year-old brought to the Emergency Department with a fractured right tibia and fibula, as well as a possible closed head injury. Jason also has type 1 diabetes mellitus, managed with insulin injections. He has been scheduled for surgical repair of his lower right leg.

● Maria Ortiz (Room 308)
Maria is an 8-year-old child who was admitted from the Emergency Department with an acute exacerbation of asthma. She has a 2-year history of asthma. Past acute exacerbation have been treated with Prelone.

● De Olp (Room 310)
De is a 6-year-old girl who entered the hospital 4 days ago. A bone marrow aspiration confirmed a diagnosis of acute lymphoblastic leukemia. She has had a lumbar puncture for assessment of cerebral spinal fluid, intrathecal chemotherapy, and placement of a Port-a-Cath for administering additional chemotherapy agents.

◆ **Floor 4: Surgery Department**

● Jason Baker
Jason begins Tuesday on the Pediatric Floor (see Room 306 above). He is then transferred to the Surgery Department and undergoes surgical repair of his leg fracture. After a period in the Post Anesthesia Care Unit (PACU), he is transferred back to the Pediatric Floor and into the same room he left earlier this morning.

■ VISITING A PATIENT

Each time you sign in for a new patient and period of care, you enter the simulation at the start of that period of care. The simulations are constructed so that you can conduct a fairly complete assessment of your patient in the first 30 minutes of each period of care. However, after completing a general survey, you should begin to focus your assessments on specific areas. For example, you should not do a head-to-toe examination each time you come into a patient's room; instead you should select assessments that are appropriate for your patient's current condition and based on how that condition is changing. Just as in the real world, a patient's data will change through time as he or she improves or deteriorates. Even if a patient remains stable, there will be diurnal variations in physiology and these will be reflected in changes in assessment data.

As soon as you sign in to begin working with a patient, a clock appears to help you keep track of time. The clock, which operates in "real time," is located in the bottom left-hand corner of the screen when you are in the Nurses' Station and in the top right-hand corner when you are in a patient's room.

To become familiar with some of the learning resources in VCE, select Maria Ortiz and choose the 0700–0829 period of care. Then click on **Nurses' Station** in the lower right corner. This procedure selects the patient and time period for your shift and sends you to a brief Case Overview. The Case Overview begins with a short video in which your preceptor asks you to review a summary on this patient. Below the video screen is a button labeled **Assignment**. Click on this button to open a summary sheet that provides information about Maria and assigns tasks for you to complete when working with this patient.

After completing the Case Overview, click on **Nurses' Station** in the lower right corner of the screen. This will take you back to the Nurses' Station, where you can begin working with your patient. Remember three things:

- You must select a patient and period of care before any of that patient's simulation and data become available to you.
- Just as in the real world, the Nurses' Station is the base from which you can access patient records and from which you go onto the floor to visit a patient.
- Before you can see another patient or access another patient's record, you must go back to the Supervisor's (Login) Computer and follow the procedure to sign out from your current period of care.

Now that you have signed in for a patient, Maria Ortiz, you have several choices. You can enter Maria's room and work with your preceptor to assess your patient. You can review Maria's patient records, including her Chart, a Kardex plan of care, her active Medication Administration Record (MAR), and the Electronic Patient Record (EPR), all of which contain data that have been collected since Maria entered the hospital. You may know that some hospitals have only paper records; others have only electronic records. Canyon View Regional Medical Center, the *VCE* virtual hospital, has a combination of paper records (the patient's Chart, Kardex, MAR) and electronic records (the EPR).

Let's begin by becoming more familiar with the Nurses' Station screen. In the upper left hand corner, find a menu with these five buttons:

- Patient Care
- Planning Care
- Patient Records
- Case Conference
- Clinical Review

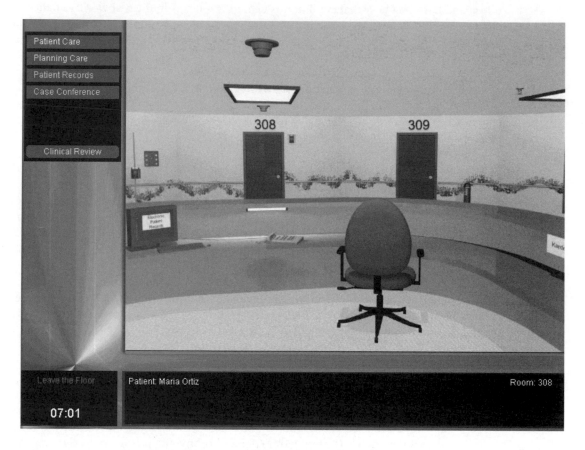

One at a time, single-click on these buttons to reveal drop-down menus with additional options for each item. First click on **Patient Care**. Two options are available for this item: **Case Overview** and **Data Collection**. You completed the Case Overview after signing in for Maria, but you can always go back to review it. For example, you might want to return there and click the **Assignment** button to review the summary of Maria's care up the start of your shift—or to remind yourself what tasks you have been asked to complete.

◆   **Data Collection**

To conduct an assessment of your patient, click **Patient Care** and then **Data Collection** from the drop-down menu. This will take you into a small anteroom (part of the patient's room) with a sink, laundry bin, and biohazards waste can. *Note:* You can also enter this anteroom by clicking on the outer door of Maria's room (Room 308). To visit your patient, complete these steps:

● First *wash your hands!* Click on the sink once to indicate you are beginning to wash. Click again to indicate you are finished washing.
● Now click on the curtain to the right of the sink and enter the patient's room.

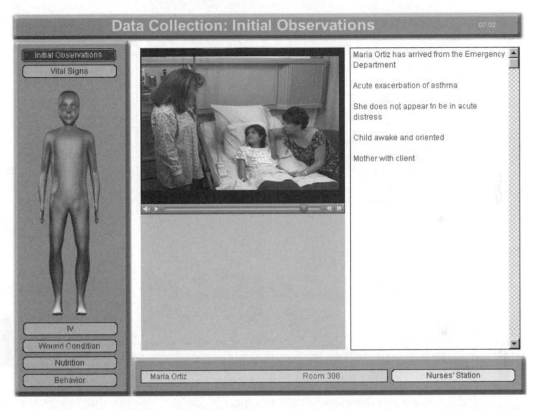

Once in the patient's room, your screen is equipped with various tools you can use for data collection. In the center of the screen, will see a still frame of your patient. Along the left side of the screen are buttons and a body model that allow you to access learning activities in which your preceptor conducts different types of assessments. Try clicking on the buttons and different body parts. (Note that the body model rotates once your cursor touches it. As you move your cursor over the model, various body parts are highlighted in orange.)

What happened when you clicked on the buttons or body parts? Many of the buttons open options for additional assessments—these always appear below the picture of your patient. Likewise, clicking on a highlighted area of the body model opens options for additional assessments. The body model serves two purposes. First, it provides a way for you to develop a sense of what assessments and physiologic systems are associated with different areas of the human body. Second, it acts as a quick navigational tool that allows you to focus on certain types of assessments.

Note that the body model is a "generic" figure without specific sexual or racial characteristics. However, we encourage you to always think about your patients as unique individuals. The body model is simply a tool designed to help you develop assessment skills by body area and navigate quickly though the simulation's learning activities. Review the diagram below to become familiar with the available Data Collection buttons and the additional options that appear when you click each button and body area.

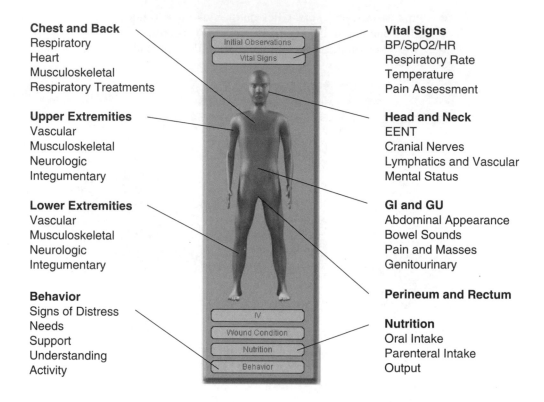

Chest and Back
Respiratory
Heart
Musculoskeletal
Respiratory Treatments

Upper Extremities
Vascular
Musculoskeletal
Neurologic
Integumentary

Lower Extremities
Vascular
Musculoskeletal
Neurologic
Integumentary

Behavior
Signs of Distress
Needs
Support
Understanding
Activity

Vital Signs
BP/SpO2/HR
Respiratory Rate
Temperature
Pain Assessment

Head and Neck
EENT
Cranial Nerves
Lymphatics and Vascular
Mental Status

GI and GU
Abdominal Appearance
Bowel Sounds
Pain and Masses
Genitourinary

Perineum and Rectum

Nutrition
Oral Intake
Parenteral Intake
Output

Whenever you click on an assessment button, either a video or still photo will be activated in the center of the screen. For some activities, data obtained during assessment are shown in a box to the right of that frame. For other assessment options, you must collect data yourself by observing the video—in these cases, no data appear in the box. You can always replay a video by simply reclicking the assessment button of the activity you wish to see again.

The *Virtual Clinical Excursions—Pediatrics* patient simulations were constructed by expert nurses to be as realistic as possible. As previously mentioned, the data for every patient change through time. During the first 30 minutes of a period of care, you will generally find that all assessment options will give you data on the patient. However, after that period, some assessments may no longer be a high priority for a patient. The expert nurses who created the patient simulations let you know when an assessment area is not a high priority by sending you a short message. These messages appear in the box on the right side of the screen, where data are normally listed. Some examples of messages you might receive include "Please rethink your priorities for assessment of this patient" and "Your assessment should be focused on other areas at this time."

To leave the patient's room, click on the **Nurses' Station** button in the bottom right-hand corner of the screen. Note that this takes you back through the anteroom, where you must wash your hands before leaving. Once you have washed your hands, click on the outer door to return to the Nurses' Station.

Now, let's review what you just learned and try a few quick exercises to get a sense of how the Data Collection learning activities become available to you. You are already signed in to care for Maria Ortiz, who entered the hospital this morning with acute exacerbations of asthma. Reenter her room from the Nurses' Station by clicking on **Patient Care** and then on **Data Collection**. You are now in the sink area of the patient's room, so wash your hands and click on the curtain to see the patient.

Start your patient care by collecting Maria's vital signs.

- Click on **Vital Signs**. Four assessment options will appear below the picture of the patient.
- Click on **BP/SpO₂/HR**. Watch the video as your preceptor measures blood pressure, oxygen saturation, and heart rate on a noninvasive multipurpose monitor. Record Maria's data for these attributes in the chart below.
- Now click on **Respiratory Rate**. This time, after a video plays, a "breathing" body model appears on the right. Measure Maria's respiratory rate by counting the respirations of the body model for the period of time your instructor recommends. Record your estimate of her respiratory rate.
- Next, click on **Temperature**. First, you will see your preceptor measuring Maria's temperature; then the thermometer reading appears in the frame to the right. Record her temperature.
- Finally, assess Maria's pain by clicking on **Pain Assessment**. Note your interpretation of Maria's pain. If she is in pain, record her pain level and characteristics.

Vital Signs	Time
Blood pressure	
SpO₂	
Heart rate	
Respiratory rate	
Temperature	
Pain rating	

Once you have collected Maria's vital signs, begin a chest examination. Point your cursor to the chest area of the body model. Click anywhere on the orange highlighted area. Four new options now appear below the picture of your patient.

- Click on **Respiratory**. Observe the video and note the data you obtain from this examination.
- Now click on **Respiratory Treatments**. How much oxygen is Maria receiving at this time?

You have now collected vital signs data and conducted a limited respiratory assessment of Maria, who was admitted with acute exacerbations of asthma. As previously mentioned, most of the assessments combine a video or still photo of the patient with data that are collected for the respective assessment. Other assessments simply provide a video, and you must collect data from the nurse-patient interaction. For example, many of the pain assessments consist of the nurse asking the patient to rate his or her pain and the patient responding with a rating. Some of the behavior assessments also require that you listen to the nurse-patient interaction and make a decision about the patient's condition, needs, or psychosocial attributes.

When you visit patients in the Well-Child Clinic and the Surgery Department, you will notice slightly different assessment options for some periods of care. However, the same types of interactions are always available. When you click on a button or area of the body model, you will be able to access a variety of patient assessments. If a video is shown, it can always be replayed by clicking on the assessment button.

■ HOW TO FIND AND ACCESS A PATIENT'S RECORDS

So far, you have visited a patient and practiced collecting data. Now you will examine the types of available patient records and learn how to access them. The records on the Pediatric Floor and in the Surgery Department include the patient Charts, Medication Administration Record (MAR), Kardex plan of care, and Electronic Patient Record (EPR). In the Well-Child Clinic, patient records are recorded only in patient charts.

You are still signed in for Maria Ortiz on the Pediatric Floor, so let's explore her records. From the Nurses' Station, each type of patient record can be accessed in two ways. Practice both methods and choose the pathway you prefer. The first option is to use the menu in the upper left corner of the screen. First, click on **Patient Records**; this reveals a drop-down menu. Then select the type of patient record you wish to review by clicking on one of these options:

- **EPR**—Electronic Patient Record
- **Chart**—The patient's chart
- **Kardex**—A Kardex plan of care
- **MAR**—The current Medication Administration Record

You can also access patient records by clicking on various objects in the Nurses' Station. On the counter inside the station you will find a set of charts, a set of Kardex plans of care, a Medication Administration Record notebook, and a computer that houses the Electronic Patient Record system. All objects inside the Nurses' Station are labeled for quick recognition.

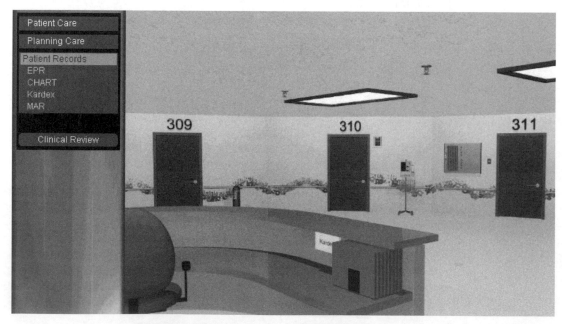

1. Chart

To open Maria's chart, click on **Chart** in the **Patient Records** drop-down menu—or click on the stack of charts inside the Nurses' Station. Colored tabs at the bottom of the screen allow you to navigate through the following sections of the chart:

- History & Physical
- Nursing History
- Admissions Records
- Physician Orders
- Progress Notes
- Laboratory Reports
- X-Rays & Diagnostics
- Operative Reports
- Medication Records
- Consults
- Rehabilitation & Therapy
- Social Services
- Miscellaneous

To flip forward in the chart, select any available tab. Once you have moved beyond the first tab (History & Physical), a **Flip Back** icon appears just above the red cross in the lower right corner. Click on **Flip Back** to return to earlier sections of the chart. The data for each patient's chart are updated during a shift; updates occur at the start of a period of care. Note that some of the records in the chart are several pages long. You will need to scroll down to read all of the pages in some sections of the chart.

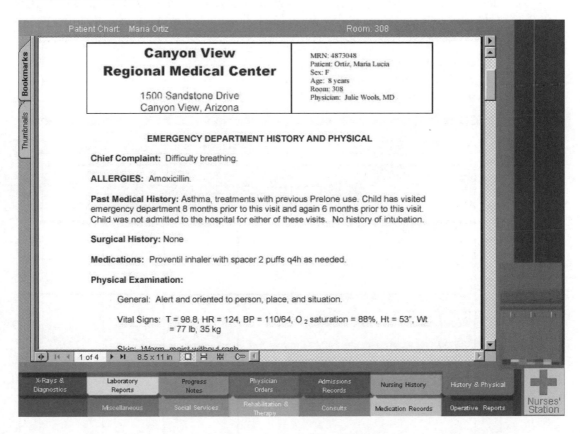

On the Pediatric Floor and in the Surgery Department, these same tabs appear in each patient's chart (see above). However, patient charts in the Well-Child Clinic have the following tabs:

- Admissions Form
- Birth & Health History
- Allergies
- Immunization Record
- Well-Child Visits
- Sick-Child Visits
- Developmental Surveillance
- Growth Charts
- Hearing & Vision Screening
- Laboratory Reports
- Referral Forms
- Anticipatory Guidance

Although the tabs differ, you navigate through the charts in the Well-Child Clinic the same way you do on the Pediatric Floor and in the Surgery Department. Flipping forward and back through the various sections is accomplished by clicking on the tabs or on the **Flip Back** icon. To close a patient's chart, click on the **Nurses' Station** icon in the lower right corner of the screen.

2. Medication Administration Record (MAR)

The notebook under the MAR sign in the Nurses' Station contains the active Medication Administration Record for each patient. This record lists the current 24-hour medications for each patient. Double-click on the MAR to open it like a notebook. (*Remember:* You can also access the MAR through the Patient Records menu.) Once open, the MAR has tabs that allow you to select patients by room number. Each MAR lists the following information for every medication a patient is receiving:

- Medication name
- Route and dosage of medication
- Time to administer medication

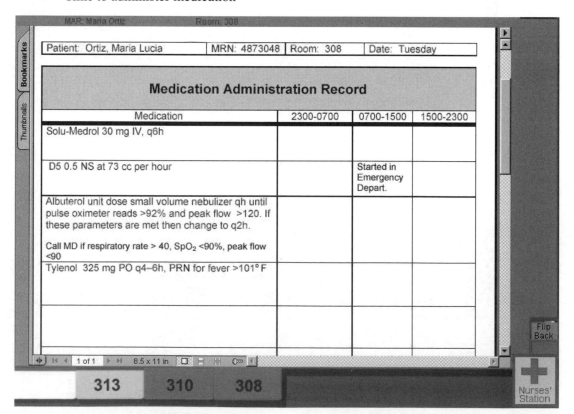

Scroll down to be sure you have read all the data. As with the patient charts, flip forward and back through the MAR by clicking on the patient room tabs or on the **Flip Back** icon. The MAR is updated at the start of every period of care. There is an MAR on the Pediatric Floor and in the Surgery Department, but not in the Well-Child Clinic. To close the MAR, click on the **Nurses' Station** icon in the lower right corner of the screen.

3. Kardex Plan of Care

Most hospitals keep a notebook in the Nurses' Station with each patient's plan of care. Canyon View Regional Medical Center's simplified plan of care is a three-page document modeled after the Kardex forms often used in hospitals. Access the Kardex through the drop-down menu (click **Patient Records**, then **Kardex**), or click on the folders beneath the Kardex sign in the Nurses' Station. Side tabs allow you to select each patient's care plan by room number. You may need to scroll down to read all of the pages.

A Flip Back icon appears in the upper right corner once you have moved past the first patient's Kardex. Use the Nurses' Station icon in the bottom right corner to return to close the Kardex.

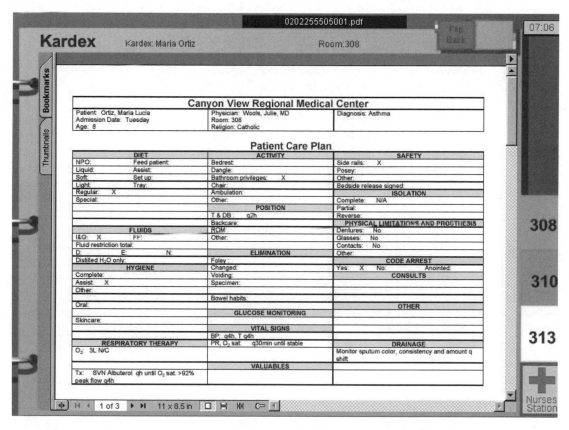

Remember: There is a Kardex on the Pediatric Floor and in the Surgery Department, but not in the Well-Child Clinic.

4. Electronic Patient Record (EPR)

Some patient records are kept in a computerized system called the Electronic Patient Record (EPR). Although some hospitals have only limited electronic patient records—or none at all—most hospitals are moving toward computerized or electronic patient record systems.

The Canyon View EPR was designed to represent a composite of commercial versions used in existing hospitals and clinics. If you have already used an EPR in a hospital, you will recognize the basic features of all commercial or custom-designed EPRs. If you have not used an EPR, the Canyon View system will give you an introduction to a very basic computerized record system.

You can use the EPR to review data already recorded for a patient—or to enter assessment data that you have collected. The EPR is continuously updated. For example, when you begin working with a patient for the 1100–1229 period of care, you have access to all the data for that patient up to 1100. The EPR contains all data collected on the patient from the moment he or she entered the hospital. The Canyon View EPR allows you to examine how data for different attributes have changed during the time the patient has been in the hospital. You may also examine data for all of a patient's attributes at a particular time. Remember, the Canyon View EPR is fully functional, as in a real hospital. Just as in real life, you can enter data during the period of care in which you are working, but you cannot change data from a previous period of care.

At Canyon View Regional Medical Center, there is an EPR system for patients on the Pediatric Floor and in the Surgery Department. The Well-Child Clinic does not have an EPR. You can access the Pediatric or Surgery EPR once you have signed in for a patient on one of those floors. Use the Patient Records menu or find the computer in the Nurses' Station with **Electronic Patient Records** on the screen. To access a patient's EPR:

- Select the EPR option on the drop-down menu (click **Patient Records**, then **EPR**) or double-click on the EPR computer screen. This will open the access screen.
- Type in the password—this will always be **nurse2b**—but **Do Not Hit Return** after entering the password.
- Click on the **Access Records** button.
- If you make a mistake, simply delete the password, reenter it, and click **Access Records**.

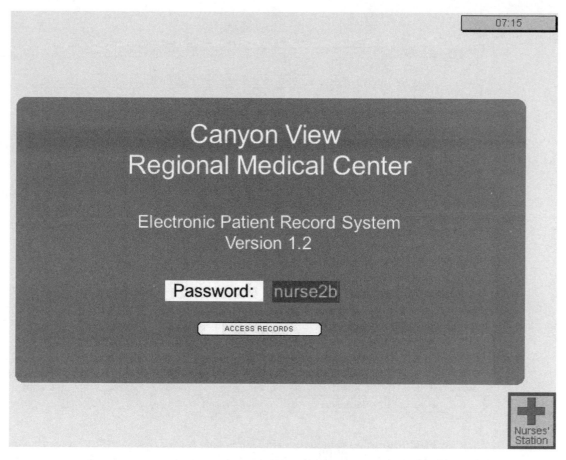

At the bottom of the EPR screen, you will see buttons for various types of patient data. Clicking on a button will bring up a field of attributes and the data for those attributes. You may notice that the data for some attributes appear as codes. The appropriate codes (and interpretations) for any attributes can be found in the code box on the far right side of the screen. Remember that every hospital or clinic selects its own codes. The codes used by Canyon View Regional Medical Center may be different from ones you have used or seen in clinical rotations. However, you will have to adjust to the various codes used by the clinical settings in which you work, so *Virtual Clinical Excursions—Pediatrics* gives you some practice using a system different from one you may already know. The different data fields available in the EPR are:

- Vital Signs
- Neurologic
- Musculoskeletal
- Respiratory
- Cardiovascular
- GI & GU
- IV
- Equipment
- Drains & Tubes
- Wounds & Dressings
- Hygiene
- Safety & Comfort
- Behavior & Activity
- Intake & Output

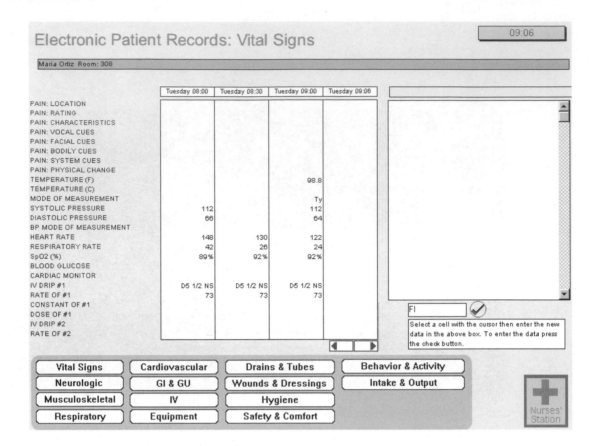

Click on **Vital Signs** and review the vital signs data for Maria Ortiz. If you want to enter data you have collected for a particular attribute (such as pain characteristics), click on the data field in which the attribute is found. (Pain characteristics are found in the Vital Signs field.) Then click on the specific attribute line, and move the highlighted box to the current time cell. Blue arrows in the lower right corner move you left and right within the EPR data fields. Once the highlighted box is in the correct time cell, type in the code for your patient's pain characteristics in the box at the lower right side of the screen, just to the left of the checkmark (√). Be sure to use the codes listed in the code box above. Once you have typed the data in this box, click on the checkmark (√) to enter them into the patient's record. The data will appear in the time cell for the attribute you have selected.

When you are ready to leave the EPR, click on the **Nurses' Station** icon in the bottom right corner of the screen.

■ PLANNING CARE

After assessing your patient, you must begin the careful process of deciding what diagnoses best describe his or her condition. For each diagnosis, you will list outcomes that you want your patient to achieve. Then, based on each outcome, you will select nursing interventions that you believe will help your patient achieve the outcomes you selected. *Virtual Clinical Excursions—Pediatrics* helps you in this process by providing a set of Planning Care resources. While you are still signed in for Maria Ortiz, click on **Planning Care** in the upper left corner of the Nurses' Station screen. You will see two options: **Problem Identification** and **Setting Priorities**.

◆ Developing Nursing Diagnoses

Click on **Problem Identification** and a note from your preceptor appears offering guidance about Maria's problems and possible diagnoses for the types of problems she may have. This diagnosis list is based on what expert nurses believe are *possible* for this particular patient. Remember, however, that not all of the diagnoses listed may apply to your patient—and that your patient may have other diagnoses that are not on the list. Your challenge and responsibility is to decide what nursing diagnoses *do* apply to your patient during each period of care. Since your patient's condition may be changing, some diagnoses may apply in one period of care but not in another. Read over the list of possible diagnoses for Maria Ortiz. When you are finished, click on **Nurses' Station** to close the Problem Identification note.

Click again on **Planning Care**. This time select **Setting Priorities**. This will open another note from your preceptor. Notice that in the third paragraph of the note, your preceptor instructs you to use the Nursing Care Matrix. This is a resource designed to help you develop nursing diagnoses for your patient. Click on **Nursing Care Matrix** at the bottom of the screen to see how. Before you can develop nursing diagnoses, you must be sure your patient actually has the characteristics of those diagnoses. It is nearly impossible for anyone to remember all of the defining characteristics for every diagnosis, so nurses consult references such as *Nursing Diagnoses: Definitions and Classification, 2001–2002* (NANDA, 2001). To make your life a little simpler and to provide training in the health informatics resources of the future, the Nursing Care Matrix provides a list of diagnoses common for your type of patient, as well as the definition for each diagnosis and the defining characteristics for each diagnosis. Ackley and Ladwig (*Nursing Diagnosis Handbook: A Guide to Planning Care*, 5th edition) have mapped specific NANDA diagnoses onto major health-illness transitions. This mapping, along with input from our expert panel of nurses, provided the list of diagnoses you see—nursing diagnoses that *might* apply to Maria Ortiz.

- Click on the first diagnosis. Note that the definition for this diagnosis now appears in a box in the upper right of the screen. The defining characteristics are listed in the box in the lower right of the screen.
- Click on another diagnosis. Review the definition and characteristics.

◆ Developing Outcomes and Interventions

For every nursing diagnosis you make, you can then select appropriate outcomes that you want your patient to achieve.

- Click on a diagnosis.
- Click on **Outcomes and Interventions** at the bottom of the screen.
- On the left-hand side of the screen, you should now see the diagnosis you selected, along with a list of the outcomes you will want your patient to achieve if she has this diagnosis.

These outcomes are based on *Nursing Outcomes Classification*, 2nd edition (Johnson, Maas, and Moorhead, 2000). This reference provides detailed lists of linkages between the NANDA diagnoses and nursing outcomes defined in the *Nursing Outcomes Classification*.

For each outcome listed, you can access a list of nursing interventions to help your patient achieve that outcome.

- Click on the first outcome.
- On the right side of your screen, you will now see lists of intervention labels in three boxes: Major Interventions, Suggested Interventions, and Optional Interventions.

Each of the intervention labels in these boxes refers to an intervention that could be implemented to help achieve the specific outcome chosen. The *Nursing Intervention Classification* system gives a label to each intervention. Therefore, the Major, Suggested, and Optional Interventions are labels, each of which has a set of nursing activities that together comprise an intervention. If you look up a label in the *Nursing Interventions Classification*, you will see that it refers to a set of different nursing activities, some or all of which can be implemented in order to achieve the desired patient outcome for that diagnosis. We used *Nursing Diagnoses, Outcomes, and Interventions: NANDA, NOC and NIC Linkages* (Johnson, Bulechek, McCloskey-Dochterman, Mass, and Moorhead, 2001) and the *Nursing Interventions Classification*, 3rd edition (McCloskey and Bulechek, 2000), to create the linkages between outcomes and interventions shown in the Nursing Care Matrix.

The Nursing Care Matrix provides you with a basic framework for learning how to move from making a diagnosis to defining patient outcomes and then to choosing the interventions you should implement to achieve those outcomes. Your instructor and the exercises in this workbook will help you develop this part of the nursing process and will provide you with more information about the nursing activities that belong with each intervention label.

■ CLINICAL REVIEW

Virtual Clinical Excursions—Pediatrics also incorporates a learning assessment system called the Clinical Review, which provides quizzes that evaluate your knowledge of your patient's condition and related conditions.

- If you are still in the Nursing Care Matrix, return to the Nurses' Station by clicking first on **Return to Diagnoses** at the bottom of the Outcomes/Interventions screen and then on **Return to Nurses' Station** at the bottom of the Diagnosis screen.
- From the menu options in the upper left corner, click on **Clinical Review**.
- You will now see a warning box that asks you to confirm that you wish to continue. Click **Clinical Review Center**.

You are now looking at the opening screen for the Clinical Review Center. Since you are working on the Pediatric Floor, you have three quiz options: **Safe Practice**, **Nursing Diagnoses**, and **Clinical Judgment**. (These same three quiz options will appear when you are working in the Surgery Department. For the Well-Child Clinic simulations, however, only the Safe Practice learning assessment is available.) Do not click on the quiz buttons yet. First, read the following descriptions of the quizzes you can select:

- **Safe Practice**
  The **Safe Practice** quiz presents you with NCLEX-RN–type questions based on the patient you worked with during this period of care. A set of five questions is randomly drawn from a pool of questions. Answer the questions, and the Clinical Review Center will score your performance.

- **Nursing Diagnoses**
  If you click on the **Nursing Diagnoses** button, you are presented with a list of 20 NANDA nursing diagnoses. You must select the five diagnoses in this list that most likely apply to your patient. The Clinical Review Center records your choices, gathers those choices that are correct, and scores your performance. The quiz then allows you

to select nursing interventions for each of the outcomes associated with NANDA diagnoses that your correctly chose. For each of your correct diagnoses, you are presented with the likely outcomes for that diagnosis; for each outcome, you will see a list of six nursing intervention labels. Only three of the intervention labels are appropriate for each outcome. You must select the correct labels. Again, your performance is automatically scored.

- **Clinical Judgement**
  The **Clinical Judgment** quiz asks you to consider a single question. This question evaluates your understanding of your patient's condition during the period of care in which you have just worked. Select your answer from four options related to your perception of your patient's stability and the frequency of monitoring you should be conducting.

On the Pediatrics Floor and in the Surgery Department, you can take one, two, or all three of the quizzes. In the Well-Child Clinic, you can only take the **Safe Practice** quiz. On any floor, when you are done with the quizzes, you must click on **Finish**. This will take you to a **Preceptor's Evaluation**, which offers a scorecard of your performance on the quizzes, discusses your understanding of the patient's condition and related conditions, and makes recommendations for you to improve your understanding.

Preceptor's Evaluation

	Correct Responses	Score
Safe Practice	3.0	18.0
Implementing Nursing Care	3.0	12.0
Clinical Judgment	0	0
Totals		30.0
Total Score	Out of 100 possible points, you received 30.0 points or 30.0%	

Preceptor's Evaluation of Clinical Review

Clincial Judgment Recommendation - We do not agree with your judgment about the client's status. Please review your assessment data and reconsider your evaluation of this patient

We want you to spend time practicing questions like those found in the Safe Practice assessment. These questions are very similar to those found on the NCLEX-RN. Also, we feel you need to study the nursing diagnoses approved by the North American Nursing Diagnosis Association (NANDA). Importantly, we want you to review the outcomes appropriate for a particular diagnosis as well as the interventions you would implement to achieve each outcome. You might want to spend time re-examining the diagnoses-outcomes-interventions linkages found in the Nursing Care Matrix. As mentioned above, the nursing diagnoses are based on approved diagnoses of the North American Nursing Diagnosis Association (NANDA). Remember that the outcomes are based on the Nursing Outcomes Classification and the interventions are based on the Nursing Interventions Classification (NIC).

Print Detailed Report   Nurses' Station

Note: We don't recommend that you take any quizzes before working with a patient. The goal of *Virtual Clinical Excursions—Pediatrics* is to help you learn and prepare for practice as a professional nurse. Reading your textbook, using this workbook to complete the CD-ROM activities, and organizing your thoughts about your patient's condition will help you prepare for the quizzes. More important, this work will help you prepare for care of real-life patients in clinical settings.

■ HOW TO QUIT OR CHANGE PATIENTS

Eventually, you will want to take a short or long break, begin caring for a different patient, or exit the software.

◆ To Take a Short Break

- Go to the Nurses' Station.
- Click on **Leave the Floor**, an icon in the lower left corner of the screen.
- You will see a screen with a variety of options.
- Click on **Break** and you will be given a 10-minute break. This stops the clock. After 10 minutes you are automatically returned to the floor, where you reenter the simulation at the same moment in time that you left.

◆ To Change Patients

Choose option 1 or option 2 below, depending on which activities you have completed during this period of care.

1. Use the following instructions *if you have already completed one or more of the quizzes* in the Clinical Review Center for your current patient:

   - Double-click on the Supervisor's (Login) Computer in the Nurses' Station.
   - Read the instructions for logging in for a new patient and period of care.
   - If you want to select a new patient on the *same* floor, click **Login**, select the new patient and period of care, and then click **Nurses' Station**.
   - If you want to work with a patient on a *different* floor, click **Return to Nurses' Station**, take the elevator to that floor, and sign in for the new patient on the Login computer in the Nurses' Station.

2. Use the following instructions *if you have* not *completed any of the quizzes* in the Clinical Review Center for your current patient:

   - Double-click on the Supervisor's (Login) Computer in the Nurses' Station.
   - Read the instructions in the Warning box. Then click on **Supervisor's Computer**.
   - The computer logs you off and gives you the option of going to the Clinical Review Center or to the Nurses' Station. Unless you wish to go to the Clinical Review Center for evaluation of the period of care you just completed, click on **Nurses' Station**.
   - Double-click on the Login Computer again, and follow the instructions to sign in for another patient. (See the third and fourth bullets in option 1 above for specific steps.)

◆ **To Quit the Software for a Long Break or to Reset a Simulation**

● From the Nurses' Station, click on **Leave the Floor** in the lower left corner of the screen.
● You will see a new screen with a variety of options.
● You may select Quit with Bookmark or Quit with Reset.
   ● **Quit with Bookmark** allows you to leave the simulation and return at the same virtual time you left. Any data you entered in the EPR will remain intact. Choose this option if you want to stop working for more than 10 minutes but wish to reenter the floor later at the exact point at which you left.
   ● **Quit with Reset** allows you to quit and reset the simulation. This option erases any data you entered in the EPR during your current session. Choose this option if you know you will be starting a new simulation when you return.

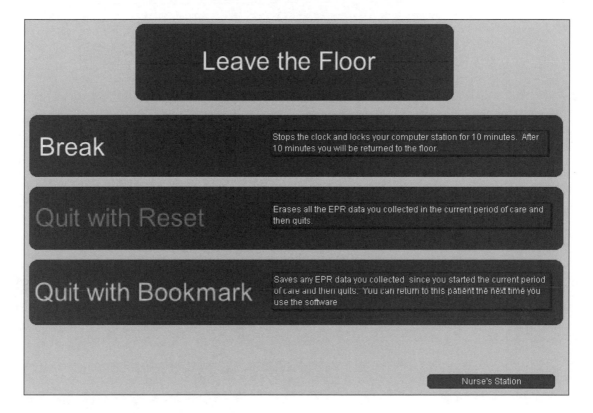

◆ **To Practice Exiting the Software**

● Click **Leave the Floor**.
● Now click **Quit with Reset**.
● A small message box will appear to confirm that you wish to quit and erase any data collected or recorded.
   ● If you have reached this message in error, click the red X in the upper right corner to close this box. You may now choose one of the other options for leaving the floor (Break or Quit with Bookmark).
   ● If you *do* wish to Quit with Reset, click **OK** on the message box.
● *Virtual Clinical Excursions—Pediatrics* will close and you will be returned to your computer's desktop screen.

A DETAILED TOUR

What do you experience when you care for patients during a clinical rotation? Well, you may be assigned one or several patients that need your attention. You follow the nursing process, assessing your patients, diagnosing each patient's problems or areas of concern, planning their care and setting outcomes you hope they will achieve, implementing care based on the outcomes you have set, and then evaluating the outcomes of your care. It is so important to remember that the nursing process is not a static, one-time series of steps. Instead, you loop through the process again and again, continuously assessing your patient, reaffirming your earlier diagnoses and perhaps finding improvement in some areas and new problems in other areas, adjusting your plan of care, implementing care as planned or implementing a revised plan, and evaluating patient outcomes to decide whether your patients are achieving expected outcomes. Patient care is hands-on, action-packed, often complex, and sometimes frightening. You must be prepared and present—physically, intellectually, and emotionally.

Textbooks help you build a foundation of knowledge about patient care. Clinical rotations help you apply and extend that book-based learning to the real world. You will know this with certainty when you experience it yourself—for example, when you first read about starting an IV but then have to start an IV on an actual patient, or when you read about the adverse effects of a medication and you then observe these adverse effects emerging in a patient. Stepping from a book onto a hospital floor seems difficult and unsettling. *Virtual Clinical Excursions—Pediatrics* is designed to help you make the transition from book-based learning to the real world of patient care. The CD-ROM activities provide you with the practice necessary to make that transition by letting you apply your book-based knowledge to virtual patients in simulated settings and situations. Each simulation was developed by an expert nurse or nurse-physician team and is based on realistic patient problems, with a rich variety of data that can be collected during assessment of the patient.

Several types of patient records are available for you to access and analyze. This workbook, the software, and your textbook work together to allow you to move from ***book-based learning*** to real-life ***problem-based learning***. Your foundational knowledge is based on what you have learned from the textbook. The *VCE—Pediatrics* patient simulations allow you to explore this knowledge in the context of a virtual hospital with virtual patients. Questions stimulated by the software can be answered by consulting your textbook or reviewing a patient simulation. The workbook is similar to a map or guide, providing a means of connecting textbook content to the practice of skills, data collection, and data interpretation by leading you through a variety of relevant activities based on simulated patients' conditions.

To better understand how *Virtual Clinical Excursions—Pediatrics* can help you in your transition, take the following detailed tour, in which you visit three different patients.

■ WORKING WITH A PEDIATRIC FLOOR PATIENT

In *Virtual Clinical Excursions—Pediatrics*, the Pediatric Floor can be visited between 0700 and 1500, but you can care for only one patient at a time and only in the following blocks of time, which we call *periods of care*: 0700–0829, 0900–1029, 1100–1229, and 1300–1429. For each clinical simulation, you will select a single patient and a period of care. When you have completed the assigned care for that patient, you can then select a new patient and period of care. You can also reset a simulation at any point and work through the same period of care as many times as you want. Each time you sign in for a patient and time period, you will enter that session at the beginning of that period of care (unless you have previously "saved" a session by choosing Break or Quit with Bookmark).

Consider, for a moment, a typical Pediatric Floor during the period between 0700 and 1500. Suppose that you could accompany a preceptor on that floor and provide care for patients during that 8-hour shift. Different expert nurses might take slightly different approaches, but almost certainly each nurse would establish priorities for patient care. These priorities would be based on report during shift change, a review of the patient records, and the nurse's own assessment of each patient.

At the beginning of a period of care, the assessment of each patient is usually accomplished by a general survey, that is, a fairly complete assessment of a patient's physical and psychosocial status. After the general survey, a nurse subsequently conducts focused assessments during the rest of the shift. The specific types of data collected in such focused assessments are determined by the nurse's interpretation of each patient's condition, needs, and applicable clinical pathways for independent and collaborative care. Depending on an agency's protocols and standards of care for the pediatric patient, a nurse may conduct more than one comprehensive assessment during a shift, with focused surveys completed between the general surveys. Regardless of individual agency protocol, any pediatric floor patient would have at least one general survey and two or more focused surveys over the period of the shift.

Now let's put these guidelines to practice by returning to the Pediatric Floor at Canyon View Regional Medical Center. This time, you will care for De Olp, a 6-year-old girl with leukemia.

1. Enter and Sign In for De Olp

- Insert your *VCE—Pediatrics* **Patients' Disk** in your CD-ROM drive and double-click on the **VCE—Pediatrics** icon on your desktop. Wait for the program to load.
- When Canyon View Regional Medical Center appears on your screen, click on the hospital entrance to enter the lobby.
- Click on the elevator. Once inside, click on the panel to the right of the door; then click on button **3** for the Pediatric Floor.
- When the elevator opens onto the Pediatric Floor, click on the **Nurses' Station**.
- Inside the Nurses' Station, double-click on the **Supervisor's (Login) Computer** and select De Olp as your patient for the 0900–1029 period of care.

2. Case Overview

- Signing in automatically takes you to the patient's Case Overview. Your preceptor will appear and speak briefly on the video screen.
- Listen to the preceptor; then click on **Assignment** below the video screen.
- You will now see a Preceptor Note, which is a summary of care for De Olp, covering the period of care just before the one you are now working.
- Review the summary of care. Scroll down to read the entire report.
- On the next page, make note of any information that you feel is important or that will require follow-up work, either with the patient or through examination of her records.

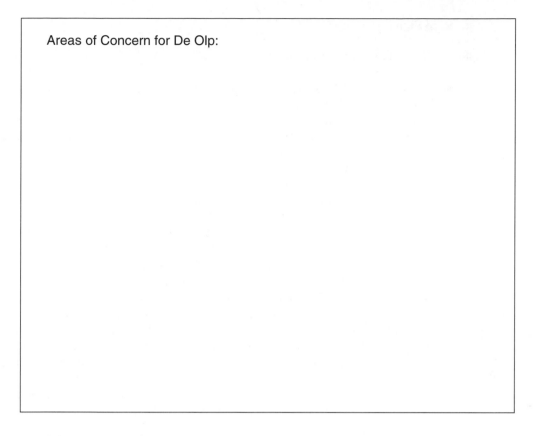

Areas of Concern for De Olp:

- When you have finished the case overview, click on **Nurses' Station** in the lower right corner of the screen and you will find yourself in the Pediatric Nurses' Station.

3. Initial Impressions

Visit your patient immediately to get an initial impression of her condition.

- On the menu in the upper left corner of your screen, click on **Patient Care**. From the options on the drop-down menu, click on **Data Collection**. *Remember:* You can also visit the patient by double-clicking on the door to her room (Room 310).
- In the anteroom, wash your hands by double-clicking on the sink. Then click on the curtain to enter the patient area.
- Inside the room, you will see many different options for assessing this patient. First, click on **Initial Observations** in the top left corner of the screen. Observe and listen to the interaction between the nurse preceptor and the patient. Note any areas of concern, issues, or assessments that you may want to pursue later.
- Now that you have gotten an initial impression of you patient, you have a few choices. In some cases, you might wish to leave the patient and access her records to develop a better understanding of her condition and what has happened since she was admitted. However, let's stay with De a while longer to conduct a few physical and psychosocial assessments.

4. Vital Signs

Obtain a full set of vital signs from De Olp.

- Click on **Vital Signs** (just below the Initial Observations button). This activates a pathway that allows you to measure all or just some of your patient's vital signs. Four options now appear under the picture of De Olp. Clicking on any of these options will begin a data collection sequence (usually a short video) in which the respective vital sign is measured. The vital signs data change over time to reflect the temporal changes you would find in a patient such as De. Try the various vital signs options to see what kinds of data are obtained.
  - First, click on **BP/SpO$_2$/HR**. Wait for the video to begin; then observe as the nurse preceptor uses a noninvasive monitor to measure De's blood pressure, SpO$_2$, and heart rate. After the video stops, the preceptor's findings appear as digital readings on a monitor to the right of the video screen. Record these data in the chart below. If you want to replay the video, simply click again on **BP/SpO$_2$/HR**. *Note:* You can replay any video in this manner—as often as needed.
  - Now click on **Respiratory Rate**. This time, after the video plays, an image of a breathing body model appears on the right. Count the respirations for the amount of time recommended by your instructor. Record your measurement below.
  - Next, click on **Temperature**. Again, a video shows the nurse preceptor obtaining this vital sign, and the result is shown on a close-up of a digital thermometer on the right side of the screen. Record this finding in the chart below.
  - Finally, click on **Pain Assessment** and observe as the nurse preceptor asks De about her pain. Note De's response in the chart below.

Vital Signs	Time
Blood pressure	
SpO$_2$	
Heart rate	
Respiratory rate	
Temperature	
Pain rating	

5. Mental Status

From some of your vital signs assessments, you should be starting to form an idea of De's mental status. However, you can check her mental status more specifically by doing the following:

- On the left side of the Data Collection screen is a body model. When you move your cursor along the body, it begins to rotate and the area beneath your cursor is highlighted in orange.
- Place your cursor on the head area of the body model and click.
- Notice that new assessment options now appear under the picture of your patient.
- Click on **Mental Status** (the bottom option of the list).
- Observe De's responses and interactions with the nurse. Then review the data, if any, that appear to the right after the video has stopped.

6. Respiratory Assessment

De Olp has received medication that may cause fluid retention. Auscultate her lungs to see whether there is any evidence of edema.

- Click on the chest area of the body model.
- Note the new assessment options that come up beneath the picture of De.
- Click on **Respiratory**.
- Observe the examination of the anterior, lateral, and posterior chest. Then review the data collected by your preceptor.
- Do you believe there is any evidence of pulmonary edema? If so, explain what data support your conclusion.
- If you were worried about fluid retention, what other assessments might you conduct?

7. Behavior

Since this is your first visit with De, you may also want to collect some psychosocial data.

- At the bottom left corner of the screen, click on **Behavior**.
- One at a time, click on each of the behavioral assessment options that appear below the picture of De.
- As you observe each assessment, take notes on the nurse-patient interactions.
- Do any of De's responses concern you?
- Does De have family support as well as nursing support?
- What other questions do you want to ask De? When might you ask these questions?

8. Chart

You have conducted your preliminary examination of De. Next, review her patient records.

- To access the patient charts, either click on the stack of charts inside the Nurses' Station or click on **Patient Records** and then **Chart** from the drop-down menu.
- De Olp's chart automatically appears since you are signed in to care for her. As described earlier in **A Quick Tour**, the chart is divided into several sections. Each section is marked by a colored tab at the bottom of the screen. To flip forward and back through the chart sections, click on the labeled tabs and on the **Flip Back** icon, respectively. Once you have moved beyond a section, the tab for that section disappears. You can move back to previous sections *only* by clicking on the **Flip Back** icon, which appears above the Nurses' Station icon in the lower right corner.
- Review the following sections of De's chart: History & Physical, Nursing History, Operative Reports, and Progress Notes.

- Based on your analyses of these records and your preliminary assessment of De, summarize key issues for this patient's care in the box below.
- When you are finished, close the chart by clicking on the **Nurses' Station** icon.

Key Issues for Patient Care:

---

9. Electronic Patient Record (EPR)

Now examine the data in De Olp's EPR.

- To access the EPR, first click **Patient Records** in the upper left corner of the screen. Then click **EPR** on the drop-down menu. *Remember:* As an alternative, you can also double-click on the EPR computer in the Nurses' Station. This computer is located to the left of the Kardex and has **Electronic Patient Records** on the screen.
- On the access screen, enter the password—**nurse2b**—and click **Access Records**.
- The EPR automatically opens to the patient's Vital Signs summary. Examine De Olp's vital signs data for the past 8 hours.
- Now click **Respiratory** (three buttons below Vital Signs). The data from assessments of De's respiratory system are now shown.
- De has been receiving a medication that may cause some fluid retention. Review the data for her lung auscultation to determine where there is any evidence of pulmonary edema. Record your findings in the box on the next page.

Lung Sounds During the Past 24 Hours:

- Click on **Cardiovascular**.
- Review data collected for edema.
- List any evidence for fluid retention as evidenced by edema.
- Make sure that if edema was observed, you note the locations and quality.
- Now, make an assessment of De's clinical status:

    a. Are any of the vital signs data you collected this morning significantly different from the baselines for those vital signs?

    Circle One: Yes   No

    b. If "Yes," which data are different?

    c. Do you have any concerns about the data collected during your respiratory assessment?

    Circle One: Yes   No

    d. If you answered "No," what data tell you the patient is stable?

    e. If you answered "Yes," what are your concerns?

10. Medication Administration Record (MAR)

- De has been taking a number of medications. Access her current MAR by double-clicking on the notebook below the MAR sign in the Nurse' Station. You can also open the MAR by clicking on **Patient Records** and then on **MAR** on the drop-down menu.
- Once the MAR notebook is open, access De's records by clicking on the tab with her room number (310) at the bottom of the screen.
- Examine the MAR and note any medications that De should be given during the period of care between 0900 and 1029. Make a list of these medications, the times they are to be administered, and any assessments you should conduct before and after giving the medications.
- Click the **Nurses' Station** icon to close the MAR.

11. Planning Care

So far, you have completed a preliminary examination of De Olp and reviewed some of her records. Now you can begin to plan her care. *Note:* Before *actually* starting a plan of care, you would conduct a more thorough assessment and a more complete review of this patient's records. However, let's continue so that you can learn how to use *Virtual Clinical Excursion's* unique and valuable Planning Care resource.

- On the drop-down menu, click **Planning Care** and then **Problem Identification**.
- Read the Preceptor Note on problem identification for De Olp and write one nursing diagnosis that you think might apply to this patient. Base you decision on your preliminary assessment and review of her records.
- Click on **Nurses' Station** to close this note.
- Click again on **Planning Care** in the upper left corner of your screen. This time, select **Setting Priorities** from the drop-down menu.
- Review the Preceptor Note on setting priorities for De.
- When you have finished, click on **Nursing Care Matrix** at the bottom of your screen.
- You will now see a list of nursing diagnoses approved by the North American Nursing Diagnosis Association (NANDA) that may apply to De's condition.
- Find the diagnosis you just identified for De. Click on this diagnosis.
- Review the nursing diagnosis definition and the defining characteristics that now appear on the right side of the screen.
- Does the definition fit your patient?
- Does your patient have the defining characteristics? If not, perhaps your assessment was not complete enough for you to make this decision. What other assessments should you conduct in order to determine whether this diagnosis applies to De Olp?
- For now, assume that your diagnosis *does* apply to De. Click on the **Outcomes and Interventions** button at the bottom of the screen.
- You now see a screen that lists nursing outcomes for your diagnosis. These are based on the Nursing Outcomes Classification. If your patient has this diagnosis, these are the outcomes you will want her to achieve.
- Some or all of these outcomes will probably apply to your patient if she does indeed have the nursing diagnosis you selected.
- Click on the first outcome, and text will appear in the three boxes on the right side of the screen. These boxes show the Major, Suggested, and Optional Interventions that could be implemented to achieve the outcome you selected, based on the Nursing Interventions Classification. *Remember:* Each entry listed in these boxes is an intervention label that represents a *set* of nursing activities that you would implement.
- Review the nursing interventions, especially those in the Major Interventions box. These are the most likely interventions you would implement to achieve the outcome you have clicked. However, you should consider all of the interventions before deciding which apply to the outcome for your patient.

- Now click on **Return to Diagnoses**. At this time, you can explore other diagnoses and their respective outcomes and interventions, or you can click **Return to Nurses' Station**.

Your work with De Olp is completed for now. To quit the software and reset a simulation:

- Go to the Nurses' Station.
- Click on **Leave the Floor** in the lower left corner of the screen.
- A screen appears with a variety of options.
- Select **Quit with Reset**, which allows you to quit and reset the simulation. This option erases any data you entered in the EPR during your current session.

■ WORKING WITH A WELL-CHILD CLINIC PATIENT

In *Virtual Clinical Excursions—Pediatrics*, the Well-Child Clinic can be visited between 0700 and 1100. You can visit three different patients, but you can visit only one child at a time. Entering the clinic and selecting a patient begins a Well-Child Clinic visit in which you work with two professional nurses, one of whom is a pediatric nurse practitioner. This time, you will care for 24-month-old Paul Parker, who is accompanied by his mother.

1. Enter and Sign In for Paul Parker

- Insert your *VCE—Pediatrics* **Patients' Disk** in your CD-ROM drive and double-click on the **VCE—Pediatrics** icon on your desktop. Wait for the program to load.
- When Canyon View Regional Medical Center appears on your screen, click on the hospital entrance to enter the lobby.
- Click on the elevator. Once inside, click on the panel to the right of the door; then click on **2** for the Well-Child Clinic.
- When the elevator arrives at the Well-Child Clinic, click on the **Nurses' Station** to enter the clinic.
- You will use only one computer at this Nurses' Station—the Supervisor's (Login) Computer. Find this computer and double-click on the screen.
- Click **Login**.

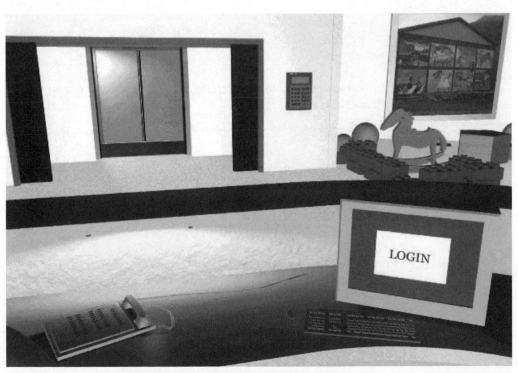

- Select Paul Parker as your patient. (*Note*: Only one period of care is available.)
- Click **Nurses' Station** in the lower right corner.

2. Case Overview

- Signing in automatically takes you to the patient's Case Overview.
- Listen to the preceptor; then click on **Assignment** below the video screen.
- Read the Preceptor Note, which summarizes important information about conducting a well-child visit and assigns specific tasks for you to complete during the visit.
- Below, note any information that you feel is important to remember when you examine a pediatric patient during a well-child visit.

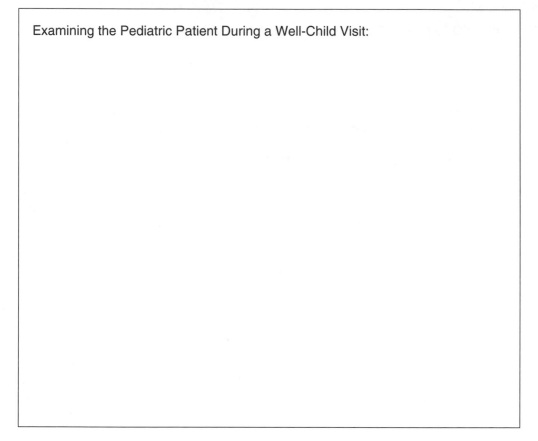

Examining the Pediatric Patient During a Well-Child Visit:

- Click on **Nurses' Station** to complete the Case Overview and return to the Well-Child Clinic Nurses' Station.

3. Preliminary Examination

Visit your patient immediately to complete a preliminary examination.

- Review the menu of options in the upper left corner of your screen.
- Click on **Physical Examination**.
- In the anteroom, double-click on the sink to wash your hands. Then click on the curtain to the right of the sink and enter the examination room.
- Click on **Preliminary Examination** at the upper left side of the screen. Notice that a list of additional assessment options for this selection appears under the picture of your patient.
- Experiment by clicking the options one at a time. After clicking each option, wait for the video to begin; then follow the professional nurse through each portion of the preliminary examination of Paul Parker.

- As you observe the assessments, make note of the types of data that are collected.
- You probably noticed that for some of the assessment options, the video does not show all of the assessments for which data appeared to the right of the video screen. Form a small collaborative group with a few of your classmates. Discuss which assessments were incomplete or missing during the preliminary examination. Identify the specific type of assessment that would yield each of the results shown to the right of the video screen. Take turns critiquing the techniques used by the nurse in the videos. Discuss what you might do differently.

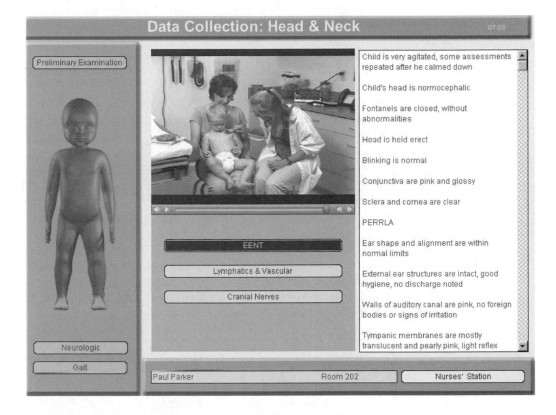

4. Other Well-Child Assessments

Now that you have observed Paul Parker's preliminary examination, conduct a physical examination of this patient by clicking on various parts of the body model. This time, you will work with the nurse practitioner. *Note:* If you receive a message telling you that the current period of care has ended (or if the clock on your screen shows that time for this visit has almost expired), go back to the Supervisor's (Login) Computer and log in for Paul Parker a second time. Simply double-click on the Login screen and follow instructions for selecting another patient—but reselect Paul Parker instead.

- First, click on the head area of the body model.
- The following assessment options appear for the head and neck area of the patient: EENT, Lymphatics & Vascular, and Cranial Nerves.
- Click on each of the options, watching the videos and examining the findings of the nurse practitioner. Describe some of the problems the nurse practitioner encounters, for example, when she tries to examine Paul's nose, mouth, and ears. Is there anything she could do differently in order to help Paul feel comfortable with an ear examination?
- Now click on the chest area of the body model.
- What types of assessment options are available?
- Watch these assessments, analyzing the data obtained from each assessment.

- Decide whether the data collected indicate any problems with Paul's respiratory or cardiovascular system. If you determined there were some problem areas, what other assessments would you want to do? What other data would you want to collect to investigate these problems in more detail?

5. Parent Interview

Now take some time to visit with Paul's mother.

- From the examination room, return to the Nurses' Station. Which button do you click to get there?
- *Remember*: You must stop to wash your hands in the anteroom.
- Once you are back in the Nurses' Station, click on **Parent Interview** (upper left side of the screen).
- On the Parent Interview screen, click on **Health Supervision** below the video monitor.
- Observe the nurse practitioner interviewing Paul's mother. Take notes on any important issues raised during these discussions.
- Now click on **Developmental Observations**.
- Again, take notes on the nurse-parent discussions.
- Based on the parent interview, how would you decide whether Paul's mother provides a safe environment for her child and follows good health supervision practices?
- How would you decide whether Paul is at the developmental stage appropriate for his age?
- Return to the Nurses' Station. This time click on the **Developmental Surveillance** button. This accesses a summary of the nurse practitioner's assessment of Paul's developmental status. Based on your examination and your observation of the parent interview, list areas in which you agree and disagree with the nurse practitioner. For example, does Paul's mother say that he does not attend day care?

Developmental Assessment Summary of Findings

Patient name: Paul Parker

Age at testing: 2 years

Date of birth: 4/15

Findings: Paul was tested in four categories today for developmental progress. These categories were motor skills, language skills, social skills and cognitive ability. In the language and cognitive skills assessment, Paul was found to be speaking frequently, but most of his words sound the same. Some phrases are understandable, and he appears to understand what is spoken to him. He follows simple commands well. According to mom, Paul is able to obey commands at home and understands what she tells him. Paul is being referred to a speech therapist at this time for evaluation of speech development progress. In the area of motor skills, Paul is doing well. He is able to walk up stairs, kick a ball, and feed himself, and he is beginning to toilet train. Socially, Paul is a shy toddler, he does not attend day care and has a sibling, age 4, at home. He is exhibiting some aggressive and selfish behavior toward his sibling. This behavior is normal for a child of Paul's age.

Impression: Paul is on target for developmental skills in cognitive, motor, and social areas and is being referred to a specialist for language development assessment.

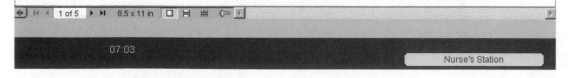

07:03

Nurse's Station

---

6. Chart

- Access Paul Parker's chart by double-clicking on the stack of charts in the Nurses' Station or by clicking **Patient Records** from the menu on the left side of the screen.
- Read the following sections of Paul's chart: Birth & Health History, Immunization Record, Well-Child Visits, Sick-Child Visits, and Growth Charts.
- Based on your analyses of these records, do you find any reasons why Paul may be sensitive about having his ears examined? List and describe other key issues for this patient's care.
- Plot Paul's length and weight on the Growth Charts. Do his measurements fall within reasonable ranges for his age?
- Are Paul's immunizations current? If not, how would you discuss with his mother the need to complete immunizations?
- Below, list any other areas that are key issues for Paul.

Key Issues for Patient Care:

Remember: The Well-Child Clinic does not have a Medication Administration Record, a Kardex plan of care, or an Electronic Patient Record. This clinic is an outpatient service provided by Canyon View Regional Medical Center, and although an EPR would be of value, the costs have prohibited its extension to the Well-Child Clinic. In an ideal setting, all patient records would be available in a computerized system, including data from every visit to the hospital or any of its associated outpatient clinics. Specifically, think about how such an EPR system would be useful to nurses in the Well-Child Clinic? How could an EPR provide data that are not already available in the chart?

It is time to leave the Well-Child Clinic. Before you can go to another floor, you must log out from your current patient:

- Double-click on the Supervisor's Computer.
- Read the Warning message that explains how to log off.
- Click on the **Supervisor's Computer** button.
- The next screen asks you whether you want to visit the Clinical Review Center (for evaluation of your work with Paul Parker) or return to the Nurses' Station.
- We want to work with a new patient now, so click **Nurses' Station**.
- Take the elevator to the Pediatric Floor and begin the next section, Working with a Perioperative Patient.

■ WORKING WITH A PERIOPERATIVE PATIENT

One of the pediatric patients at Canyon View Regional Medical Center, Jason Baker, has a badly fractured leg.

- On the Pediatric Floor, sign in to visit Jason for his Preoperative Interview.
- The interview takes place in Jason's room, so click on **Patient Care** and then **Data Collection** on the drop-down menu.
- Wash your hands, enter the room, and click **View Interview**.
- After observing the interview, click on **Summary** and read the Preceptor Note.
- Now return to the Nurses' Station and sign out so that you can go to the Surgery Department, where Jason has been transported for Preoperative Care.
- Take the elevator to the 4th floor. Click on the Nurses' Station and sign in to visit Jason during his preoperative care.
- Although you cannot observe Jason's surgery, you can see him now in the Preoperative Care Bay and later in the PACU
- Once Jason is transferred out of PACU, you can visit him in his room on the Pediatric Floor.

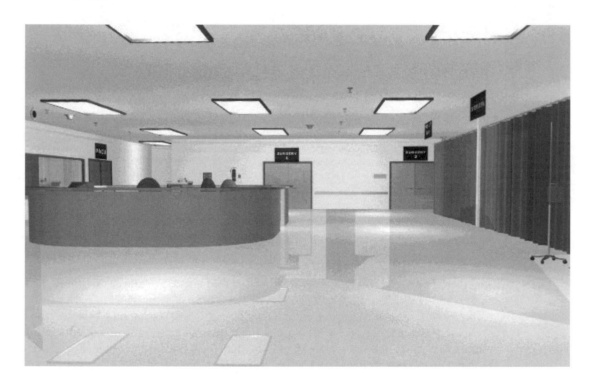

● Spend some time in each of the different perioperative settings described on p. 42. Then compare these perioperative settings with the settings on the Pediatric Floor and in the Well-Child Clinic. Use the following chart and focus your comparisons on the themes listed in the left column.

Comparison of Settings in Canyon View Regional Medical Center			
Activities and Resources	Perioperative Settings	Pediatric Floor Settings	Well-Child Clinic Settings
Patient Assessments			
Planning Care			
Types of Patient Records			

Remember: *Virtual Clinical Excursions—Pediatrics* is designed to provide a realistic learning environment. Within Canyon View Regional Medical Center, you will not necessarily find the same type of patient records, clinical settings, Nurses' Station layout, or hospital floor architecture that you find in your real-life clinical rotations. If you have already had experience within actual clinical settings, take a few moments to list the similarities and differences between the Canyon View virtual hospital and the real hospitals you have visited. There is considerable variation among hospitals in the United States, so think of *Virtual Clinical Excursions—Pediatrics* as simply one type of hospital and take advantage of the opportunity to practice learning how, where, when, and why to find the information, medication, and equipment resources you need to provide the highest quality patient care.

The following icons are used throughout the workbook to help you quickly identify particular activities and assignments:

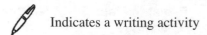 Indicates a reading assignment—tells you which textbook chapter(s) you should read before starting each lesson

Indicates a writing activity

Marks the beginning of an interactive CD-ROM activity—signals you to open or return to your *Virtual Clinical Excursions—Pediatrics* Patients' Disk

Indicates a continuation of CD-ROM instructions

Indicates questions and activities that require you to consult your textbook

LESSON 1

Growth and Development

👓 **Reading Assignment:** Developmental Influences on Child Health Promotion (Chapter 5)
Health Promotion of the Infant and Family (Chapter 10)

Patient: Matthew Brown, Room 205

This lesson will acquaint the learner with aspects of infant growth and development, as well as some of the major milestones of this age group.

💿 **CD-ROM Activity**

Begin by going to the Well-Child Clinic on Floor 2 of the hospital. Enter the Nurses' Station, double-click on the **Supervisor's (Login) Computer**, and sign in to work with Matthew Brown in Room 205. Once you are signed in and have completed the Case Overview, access Matthew's Chart by clicking on **Patient Records** in the drop-down menu on the left side of the screen. (*Remember:* You can also access these patient records by clicking on the stack of charts on the Nurses' Station desktop.) Click on the **Developmental Surveillance** tab and review this section of his Chart.

✒️ **Writing Activity**

1. According to the summary of findings, Matthew's father reports that the child demonstrates some anxiety related to adults who are not close family members. (*Hint:* You can learn more about anxiety in Table 10-2 in your textbook.)

    a. Define stranger anxiety.

    b. Identify how you would modify Matthew's plan of care in relation to testing for developmental milestones to minimize stranger anxiety.

Now conduct a complete physical assessment of your patient. Return to the Nurses' Station and click on **Physical Examination** on the drop-down menu. After you wash your hands and enter Matthew's room, click on **Preliminary Examination** and observe the nurse and the nurse practitioner as they collect data pertaining to Matthew. Make sure you also click on each of the six body areas on the 3-D body model. When you are finished, return to the Nurses' Station and click on **Parent Interview**. Watch both segments of the interview (by clicking the two options below the video screen), but pay special attention to the Developmental Observations segment.

 2. Identify three milestones in the gross motor skill area that a child Matthew's age should have achieved. What specific examples of gross motor skills did you observe during the parent interview or physical examination? (*Hint:* For more information on gross motor skills, see Table 10-2 in your textbook.)

3. Describe Matthew's language abilities at this age as reported by his father and as observed on the videos.

 4. Matthew's father asks what he should expect to see happen within the next 2 months in relation to Matthew's language development. What specific counseling can you provide to answer his question? (*Hint:* If you need assistance, refer to Table 10-2 in your textbook.)

5. List five fine motor skills that a 10-month-old child should have mastered. List specific examples of fine motor skills that Matthew demonstrated during the parent interview or the physical examination.

Five fine motor skills a 10-month-old child should have mastered	Fine motor skills Matthew demonstrated

6. According to Erikson's theory of psychosocial development, a child of Matthew's age is in what stage of development? (*Hint:* To review theories of psychosocial development, refer to Chapter 10 of your textbook.)

7. Describe the primary features of this stage of development.

 Leave Matthew's room. (*Remember:* You must wash your hands first.) Return to the Nurses' Station and click on **Developmental Surveillance** on the drop-down menu. Briefly review the Developmental Assessment Summary Findings.

8. Define the concept of object permanence and give a specific example of Matthew's behavior or reported behavior that reflects this concept.

On the following page, review the CDC growth chart entitled "Birth to 36 Months: Boys—Length-for-Age and Weight-for-Age Percentiles."

Birth to 36 months: Boys
Length-for-age and Weight-for-age percentiles

NAME _____

RECORD # _____

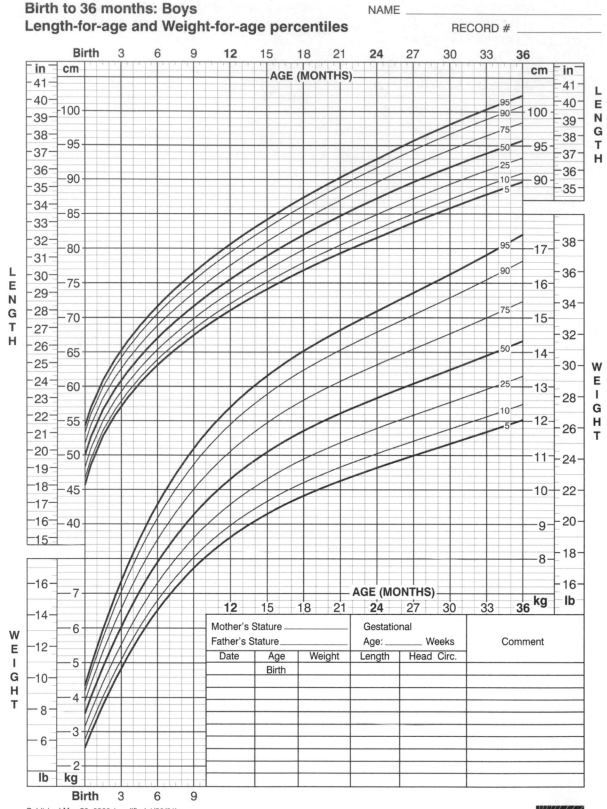

Published May 30, 2000 (modified 4/20/01).
SOURCE: Developed by the National Center for Health Statistics in collaboration with
the National Center for Chronic Disease Prevention and Health Promotion (2000).
http://www.cdc.gov/growthcharts

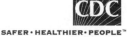

SAFER · HEALTHIER · PEOPLE™

9. Plot Matthew's weight on the growth chart on the previous page. Matthew is at the _____ percentile for weight at 10 months of age. What is the significance of this finding?

On the following page, review the CDC growth chart entitled "Birth to 36 Months: Boys—Head Circumference-for-Age and Weight-for-Length Percentiles."

**Birth to 36 months: Boys
Head circumference-for-age and
Weight-for-length percentiles**

NAME _____

RECORD # _____

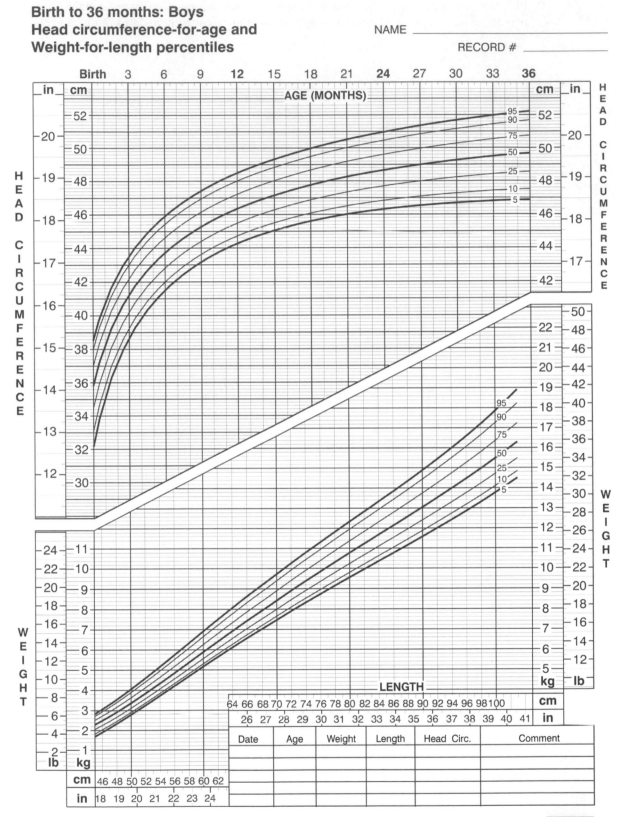

Date	Age	Weight	Length	Head Circ.	Comment

Published May 30, 2000 (modified 10/16/00).
SOURCE: Developed by the National Center for Health Statistics in collaboration with
the National Center for Chronic Disease Prevention and Health Promotion (2000).
http://www.cdc.gov/growthcharts

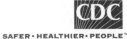

SAFER · HEALTHIER · PEOPLE™

10. Plot Matthew's head circumference on the growth chart on the previous page. He is at the
_____ percentile for head growth at 10 months. What is the significance of this finding?

11. Matthew has eight deciduous teeth. His father asks what he can do to decrease the pain
associated with teething. What specific behavior(s) did you observe on the physical assessment videos that suggest evidence of Matthew teething? Replay the videos if necessary.
(*Hint:* To learn more about teething, consult textbook Chapter 10.)

12. Play is an important part of infant development and exploration. List three safe toys that
would be appropriate for Matthew's father to use for play and for development of visual,
auditory, and tactile senses. (*Hint:* Consult Table 10-1 in your textbook.)

Visual

Auditory

Tactile

LESSON 2

History and Physical Assessment

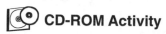 **Reading Assignment:** Communication and Health Assessment of the Child and Family (Chapter 6)
Physical and Developmental Assessment of the Child (Chapter 7)
Health Promotion of the Newborn and Family (Chapter 8)
Health Problems of the Newborn (Chapter 9)
Health Promotion of the Infant and Family (Chapter 10)

Patient: Matthew Brown, Room 205

This lesson will acquaint the learner with salient aspects of the history and physical assessment of a 10-month-old well child. The learner will review possible techniques for performing a physical assessment of a child and what some of the important findings represent at this age. Anticipatory guidance issues will be presented as they relate to the child's status in the existing family structure.

 CD-ROM Activity

To begin this exercise, go to the Well-Child Clinic on Floor 2 and enter the Nurses' Station. Locate the Login Computer and sign in to work with Matthew Brown in Room 205. Once you have signed in, return to the Nurses' Station and open Matthew's Chart by clicking on **Patient Records** on the drop-down menu. Now click on the **Birth & Health History** tab. Review this section, paying particular attention to Matthew's Prenatal and Birth History Information and his Health History. (*Note:* You will need to scroll down to read the Health History.)

✎ **Writing Activity**

1. What is the purpose of obtaining a birth history for a 10-month-old infant?

2. Identify any perinatal problems or events that might have an impact on Matthew's current health status.

→ Return to Matthew's Chart and review the forms provided in the following sections: Well-Child Visits and Sick-Child Visits.

3. Briefly describe Matthew's health status from birth to the current time.

4. What was Matthew's temperature at the sick-child visit 1 month ago? What is the clinical significance of this finding in a child his age? (*Hint:* See the inside back cover of your textbook for body temperature norms.)

5. What might possibly account for Matthew's heart rate at this sick visit?

→ Click on **Hearing & Vision Screening** in Matthew's Chart. Review the Hearing and Vision Screening Form for Children Under 3 (scroll down to page 2). Then click on **Laboratory Reports** and review the Newborn Screening Test Results for Matthew.

6. Based on the results of these tests and the family history of illness, should the practitioner discuss other possible testing for Matthew at this time? If so, what type(s) of testing? (*Hint:* For more information on inborn errors of metabolism, see textbook Chapter 9; to learn more about auditory testing practices, see Chapter 7.)

7. When is the most appropriate time to conduct the newborn screening test for PKU? (*Hint:* If you need assistance, refer to the section on Newborn Screening for Disease in Chapter 8.) Choose one:

    a. Within 2 to 4 hours of the newborn's birth
    b. Anytime prior to discharge from the hospital
    c. After 24 hours of life and prior to discharge from the hospital

8. What did the practitioner recommend Matthew be given for an elevated temperature? Based on his weight at the time of the visit, what dosage should Matthew's father be directed to administer? (*Hint:* Information on controlling elevated temperatures can be found in Chapter 27 of your textbook.)

 9. What would be the best way to obtain a nutritional assessment for Matthew? (*Hint:* Review nutritional assessment in Chapter 6 of your textbook.)

→ Return to the Nurses' Station and enter Matthew Brown's room (Room 205) to conduct a complete physical examination. One at a time, click on **Preliminary Examination, Neurologic**, and **Gait**. For each of these areas, observe the videos and review the data collected by clicking on each of the assessment options that appear under the video screen. When you are finished, complete these same steps for each of the six body areas on the 3-D model.

10. Given Matthew's chronologic age and your knowledge of stranger fear, identify an appropriate approach for conducting a review of systems physical examination that would cause the least amount of protest and more cooperation on his part. What approach does the nurse in the video use for examining Matthew?

11. What distraction techniques does the nurse use while performing the physical examination?

12. How does the nurse evaluate Matthew's hearing during the preliminary examination?

 Questions 13–18 are related to discussions from Chapter 7 of the textbook.

13. How does the nurse test Matthew's red reflex? What is the significance of the red reflex?

14. Which one of the following does the nurse use to evaluate Matthew's tympanic membranes?
    a. Otoscope
    b. Stethoscope
    c. Ophthalmoscope

15. While assessing Matthew's respiratory status, you note that his breathing at this age is primarily:
    a. diaphragmatic.
    b. abdominal.
    c. intercostal.

16. Matthew's heart rate at the time of this visit is approximately 125 beats per minute. In addition to auscultating for a murmur, what other physical signs might you evaluate to ascertain normal cardiac functioning?

17. What technique does the nurse use to examine Matthew's liver? Where should the liver be found in a child this age?

18. How does the nurse evaluate the neurologic status of Matthew's lower extremities? What is the significance of the nurse's findings? (*Hint:* More information on neurologic assessments can be found in Chapter 7 and in Table 8-4 of your textbook.)

Health Promotion

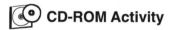 **Reading Assignment:** Communication and Health Assessment of the Child and Family (Chapter 6)
Health Promotion of the Infant and Family (Chapter 10)
Pediatric Variations of Nursing Interventions (Chapter 22)

Patient: Matthew Brown, Room 205

In this lesson the learner will review important aspects of infant immunization. The learner will also describe important health promotion aspects appropriate for an older infant in relation to parent teaching for illness prevention and safety promotion.

CD-ROM Activity

Go to the Nurses' Station on Floor 2, click on the **Login Computer**, and sign in to work with Matthew Brown in Room 205. After the Case Overview, watch the Parent Interview (click on **Parent Interview** in the upper left corner of the Nurses' Station screen). When the interview is over, return to the Nurses' Station. Click on **Patient Records** to access Matthew's Chart. First review the history and physical examination data in the Well-Child visits section of the Chart. Then click the **Flip Back** icon to open and review Matthew's Immunization Record.

 Questions 1 through 9 deal with information discussed in the Immunization section of Chapter 12 in your textbook.

1. Matthew's father should be informed that three immunizations will be necessary at Matthew's next visit. Identify these immunizations.

   a.

   b.

   c.

2. During the Parent Interview what does Matthew's father say about the foods Matthew eats? What anticipatory guidance is appropriate to give the father regarding Matthew's food intake and prevention of choking?

Birth to 36 months: Boys
Length-for-age and Weight-for-age percentiles

NAME _____

RECORD # _____

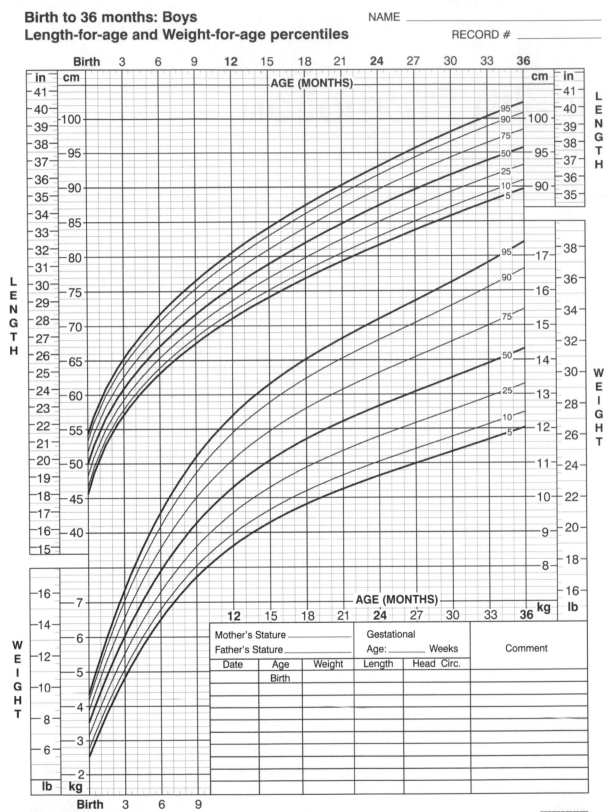

Published May 30, 2000 (modified 4/20/01).
SOURCE: Developed by the National Center for Health Statistics in collaboration with
the National Center for Chronic Disease Prevention and Health Promotion (2000).
http://www.cdc.gov/growthcharts

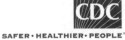

SAFER · HEALTHIER · PEOPLE™

3. Matthew's father is concerned that Matthew sometimes has a low-grade fever with a cold. Based on Matthew's weight (see CDC growth chart on p. 60), what is an appropriate dose of acetaminophen (Tylenol)? (*Hint:* Refer to Table 27-4 in your textbook if you need assistance.)

4. What information does the nurse discuss regarding Matthew's activity and safety around the home? In addition to the precautions that Matthew's father mentions, what other anticipatory guidance would you provide regarding home safety?

5. Describe two interventions that Matthew's father may perform just before their next clinic visit to reduce the pain of immunizations. (*Hint:* Review in your textbook the Atraumatic Care box on p. 534 and the discussion on immunization reactions in Chapter 12.)

   a.

   b.

6. At the next clinic visit, just before Matthew receives his immunizations, what specific information should his father be given? (*Hint:* For more information on immunization administration, see Chapter 12 in your textbook.)

7. On the blank immunization record below, enter the necessary information the nurse should document each time a child receives an immunization. A sample vaccine label is provided for reference. The VIS data is 9/98.

Sample label:

Prevnar (pneumococcal 7-valent conjugate vaccine) (diptheria CRM197 protein)

Manufacturer: Lederle Laboratories Division, NY

Lot #234-123   Expires 2/02/05

Keep refrigerated

Patient name: _____

Birthdate: _____

Vaccine administrator: Make sure you give the parent/guardian all appropriate Vaccine Information Statements (VIS) and an updated shot record at every visit.

Vaccine and route (circle type given)	Date given	Site given (LA, RA, LT, RT)	Vaccine lot number	Vaccine manufacturer	VIS date*	Signature or initials of vaccine administrator	Comments
Hepatitis B - 1 ____ mcg (IM)							
Hepatitis B - 2 ____ mcg (IM)							
Hepatitis B - 3 ____ mcg (IM)							
DTaP • DT • Td - 1 (IM)							
DTaP • DT • Td - 2 (IM)							
DTaP • DT • Td - 3 (IM)							
DTaP • DT • Td - 4 (IM)							
DTaP • DT • Td - 5 (IM)							
DTaP/Hib - 4 (IM)							

8. On the figure below indicate with an **X** the most appropriate site(s) for Matthew to receive his next three immunizations.

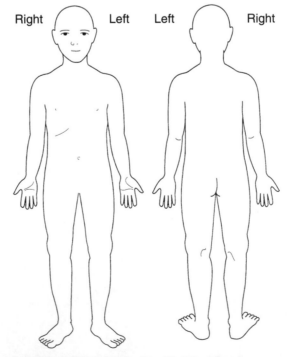

Right   Left   Left   Right

Refer to textbook Chapters 12 and 14 to learn more about dental health and fluoride.

9. What anticipatory guidance is appropriate in relation to dental development in a 10-month-old child?

➤ In the Sick-Child Visits section of Matthew's Chart, review the form for his sick-child visit at 9 months of age. Then click on the **Flip Back** icon until you have reached the Well-Child Visits tab. Review the section on sleep.

10. What information can you gather and synthesize from this history that could have an impact on Matthew's dental/oral health?

11. What preventive measures could Matthew's father take to decrease the likelihood of dental caries and otitis media? (*Hint:* For more information on dental health, see Chapters 12 and 14 in your textbook; for more information on otitis media, see Chapter 32.)

➤ Close Matthew's Chart and visit his room to observe his preliminary examination. (*Remember:* From the Nurses' Station, click on **Physical Examination**. This takes you to the anteroom. Wash your hands, click on the curtain to enter Matthew's room, and then click on **Preliminary Examination**.)

12. a. What is Matthew's current weight?

   b. Describe the car safety issues most appropriate for Matthew's father to consider in regard to the proper type, use, and placement of car seat and safety restraint. (*Hint:* To learn more about motor vehicle injuries, consult textbook Chapters 12 and 14.)

13. List three preventive measures that Matthew's father can take to prevent injuries in each of the following areas.

    a. Suffocation/drowning:

    b. Falls:

    c. Poisoning:

    d. Aspiration:

    e. Burns:

➤ Return to the Nurses' Station and review the Parent Interview video.

14. During the interview, the nurse asks the father about Matthew's outside environment and certain materials. Identify the specific question the nurse asks.

15. What specific concern regarding the materials mentioned in question 14 should be further explored? Provide the rationale for such guidance. (*Hint:* If you need help, refer to p. 675 in the textbook.)

LESSON **4** _____

Growth and Development

_____

✍ **Reading Assignment:** Physical and Developmental Assessment of the Child (Chapter 7)
Health Promotion of the Toddler and Family (Chapter 12)
Impact of Cognitive or Sensory Impairment on the Child and Family (Chapter 19)

Patient: Paul Parker, Room 202

This lesson will acquaint the learner with aspects of toddler growth and development and psychosocial development, as well as some major milestones of this age group.

💿 **CD-ROM Activity**

Go to the Nurses' Station, click on the **Login Computer**, and sign in to work with Paul Parker. Access Paul's records by clicking on the stack of charts on the Nurses' Station desktop or by clicking **Patient Records** from the drop-down menu on the left side of the screen. In the Chart, click on the **Developmental Surveillance** tab and review that section. (*Hint:* You can take the shortcut to this section by simply clicking **Developmental Surveillance** on the drop-down menu.) When you are finished, return to the Nurses' Station, click on **Parent Interview**, and observe the Health Supervision and Developmental Observations segments. Review Paul's developmental progress over time.

1. Are there any areas that cause you to be concerned about Paul's development? If so, what specific concerns do you have? (*Hint:* If you are not sure, return to the Developmental Assessment Summary of Findings in his Chart.)

→ In Paul's Chart, review the following sections: Birth & Health History, Sick-Child Visits, and Referral Forms. Then return to the Nurses' Station, click on **Developmental Surveillance**, and review again, if necessary.

2. Based on Paul's history, what is the most likely cause of the developmental problem?

→ Return to Paul's Chart and click on **Anticipatory Guidance**. Review this and other sections, as necessary, to answer the following questions.

3. What developmental interventions are necessary for Paul at this time?

4. What suggested activities could be discussed with Paul's parents at this time?

5. Has Paul completed other developmental tasks appropriate for his age? Give specific examples to support your answer. (*Hint:* If you need help, review the Developmental Surveillance section in the Chart. Also, read the Development section of Chapter 12 in your textbook.)

6. The toddler period is characterized by discovery of gross and fine motor skills. What major gross motor skill does Paul demonstrate that is characteristic of this stage of development?

7. Describe the toddler period according to Erikson. (*Hint:* For a refresher on Erikson's theories, read the Development Assessment section of Chapter 12 in your textbook.)

8. What does Erikson call the period described in question 7?

9. What important tasks should be accomplished during this period? (*Hint:* Read the development section of Chapter 14.)
   a. Differentiation of self from others
   b. A sense of accomplishment
   c. Ability to stand delayed gratification
   d. A and C
   e. B and C
   f. All of the above

10. How might you further assess Paul's sense of autonomy? Develop at least two questions that could be used to assess this stage of development. (*Hint:* Read the growth and development section of Chapter 12.)

11. According to Piaget, in what phase of development is Paul presently?

12. Describe this phase of development according to Piaget's cognitive theory.

13. Develop three assessment strategies that could be used to further assess Paul's phase of cognitive development.

    a.

    b.

    c.

14. During the Parent Interview, Paul's mother says she has started toilet training with Paul. How do you assess for toilet training readiness in a child this age? (*Hint:* If you need help, review the toilet training discussion in Chapter 12 in your textbook.)

15. Paul's mother expresses a specific concern regarding his behavior. What anticipatory guidance can you provide her related to this concern in a 24-month-old child?

→ Return to the Nurses' Station and click on **Patient Records** in the drop-down menu. Review the Growth Charts section.

16. On the growth chart on the following page, plot Paul's head circumference at:

   a. 12 months of age

   b. 24 months of age

Birth to 36 months: Boys
Head circumference-for-age and
Weight-for-length percentiles

NAME _____

RECORD # _____

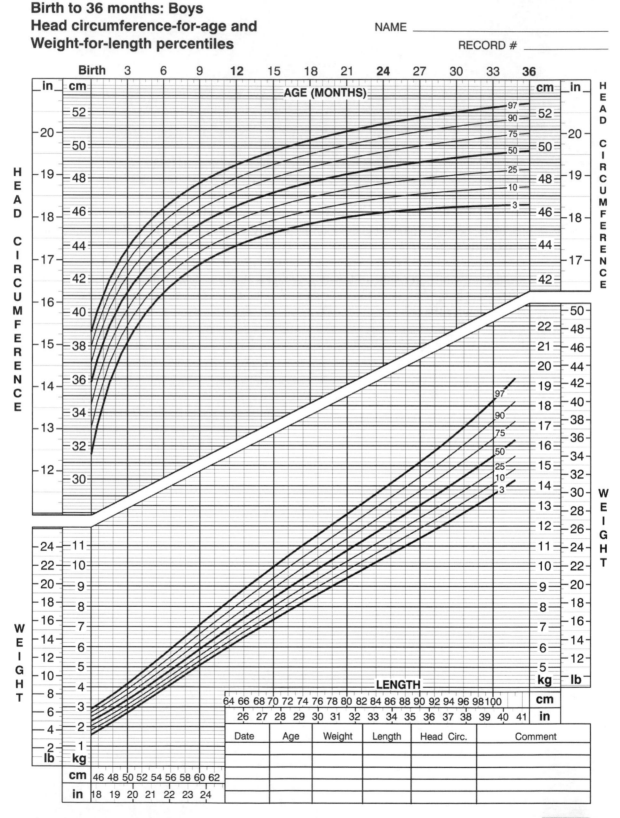

Date	Age	Weight	Length	Head Circ.	Comment

SOURCE: Developed by the National Center for Health Statistics in collaboration with
the National Center for Chronic Disease Prevention and Health Promotion (2000).
http://www.cdc.gov/growthcharts

17. Is there any cause for concern regarding Paul's head growth? Give specific reasons for your answer.

18. Plot Paul's present weight and height on the growth chart on the following page. (*Hint:* Refer to Paul's Chart for these data.)

Birth to 36 months: Boys
Length-for-age and Weight-for-age percentiles

NAME _____

RECORD # _____

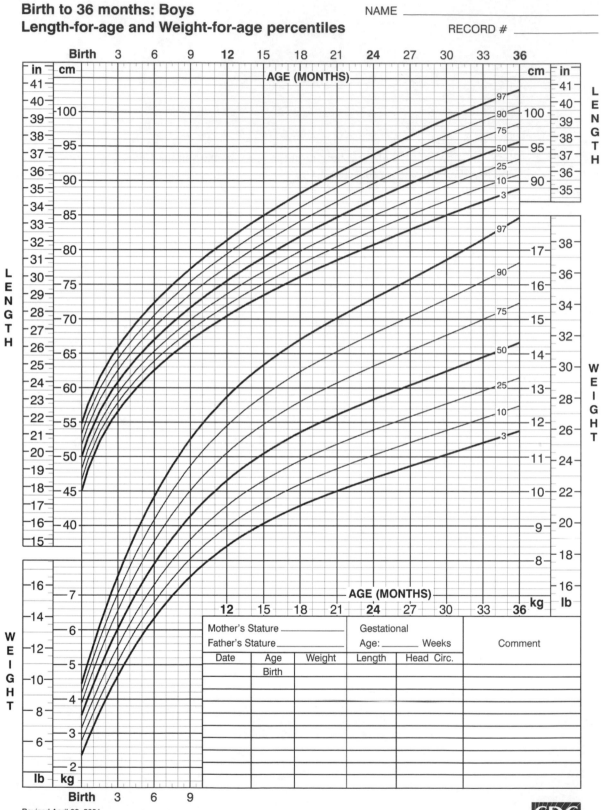

Revised April 20, 2001.
SOURCE: Developed by the National Center for Health Statistics in collaboration with
the National Center for Chronic Disease Prevention and Health Promotion (2000).
http://www.cdc.gov/growthcharts

19. What is the average weight and height for a 2-year-old child? (*Hint:* Review promoting growth and development in Chapter 12.)

20. Approximately how much body weight is gained on average per year during the toddler period?

21. Play is essential during the toddler years for promoting continued development. Give examples of play activities that promote physical, social, and mental development. (*Hint:* If you need assistance, refer to Chapter 14 in your textbook and review Paul's Chart.)

Physical

Social

Mental

History and Physical Assessment

Reading Assignment: Physical and Developmental Assessment of the Child (Chapter 7)
Health Problems of Newborns (Chapter 9)
Health Promotion of the Toddler and Family (Chapter 12)
Impact of Cognitive or Sensory Impairment on the Child and Family (Chapter 19)
The Child with Respiratory Dysfunction (Chapter 23)
The Child with Integumentary Dysfunction (Chapter 30)

Patient: Paul Parker, Room 202

This lesson will familiarize the learner with the essential aspects of the history and physical assessment of a 24-month-old well child. The learner will review possible techniques for performing a physical assessment of a child and what some of the important findings represent at this age. Anticipatory guidance issues will be presented as they relate to the child's status in the existing family structure.

CD-ROM Activity

Begin this exercise by going to the Nurses' Station of the Well-Child Clinic (Floor 2). Locate the Login Computer and sign in to work with Paul Parker. After watching the Case Overview, return to the Nurses' Station and access Paul's Chart by clicking on **Patient Records** from the drop-down menu. Inside his Chart, click on the **Birth & Health History** tab and read this section. Then click on **Sick-Child Visits** and review the forms from Paul's visits to the clinic.

1. Were any significant findings documented in the Birth History section? If so, please describe each finding below.

2. Explain the significance of newborn hyperbilirubinemia and the cause(s) for this condition. (*Hint:* For more information on hyperbilirubinemia, consult Chapter 9 in your textbook.)

3. Paul had several other illnesses during the first 2 years of life. Describe these problems below, including age of onset and the treatment plan for each problem.

Age of Onset	Problem	Treatment

4. Which sign(s) and symptom(s) of otitis media did Paul present with?
   a. Runny nose
   b. Fever
   c. Pulling at ear
   d. Fussiness
   e. All of the above

5. Based on your review, has Paul ever had an effusion associated with his ear infection? Why is an effusion a health concern?

6. Paul was diagnosed with chronic otitis media. Below, compare acute otitis media with chronic otitis media.

Acute Otitis Media

Chronic Otitis Media

 Now click on **Referral Forms** in Paul's Chart and review these forms.

 7. What factors may predispose a child to otitis media? (*Hint:* For more information on otitis media, refer to Chapter 23 of your textbook.)

8. What vaccine has reduced the incidence of otitis media in children over 2 years of age? Why is this vaccine *not* helpful in preventing infections in younger children?

9. At 20 months of age, Paul was seen in the clinic for a sick visit. Describe his illness and then differentiate the clinical findings between croup and laryngotracheobronchitis. (*Hint:* To learn more about croup syndromes, consult Chapter 23 in your textbook.)

10. What important vital sign is missing from Paul's Chart that could assist you in determining the appropriate treatment for him? (Return to the Chart if needed.)

→ In Paul's Chart, click on the **Sick-Child Visits** tab and review the form for his visit at 17 months of age.

11. Has Paul received the varicella vaccination? When did he receive it? Provide the rationale for the impression found on the Sick-Child Visit form written by the NP. (*Hint:* You may want to review the Immunization Record in Paul's Chart.)

Now review the form for Paul's sick-child visit at 6 months of age.

12. Describe the clinical findings of Paul's sick-child visit when he was 6 months old.

 13. List the common causes of diaper dermatitis and describe appropriate management strategies. (*Hint:* For guidance on skin disorders, refer to Chapter 30 in your textbook.)

Causes of Diaper Dermatitits

Appropriate Management Strategies

14. What was used to treat Paul's dermatitis? Describe how the combination of these drugs is effective in treating diaper dermatitis.

Click on **Hearing & Vision Screening** in Paul's Chart and review the forms completed for those screening tests.

15. Describe the findings of Paul's 23-month-old hearing test. What were the results? With these findings, why would he be having speech problems?

16. What were the results of Paul's vision screening examination? Is this a normal or abnormal finding?

17. What kind of test was used to examine Paul's vision in the past? Describe this test. Was the test appropriate for Paul's age at the time?

Go to the Nurses' Station. On the drop-down menu, click on **Physical Examination**. Enter Paul's room and observe the complete physical assessment. Afterward, return to the Nurses' Station, open Paul's Chart, and review the findings in the Well-Child Visits section.

 18. Based on your observation of Paul's vital signs assessment, were his vital signs within normal limits for his age? If not, what parameters were abnormal for a child of this age? (*Hint:* Look on the inside back cover of your textbook for help.)

19. Describe what techniques the nurse practitioner used in the video to assess the following areas on Paul. Also list the data obtained. Circle any abnormal data.

	Techniques	**Data**
Head		
Eyes		
Ears		
Mouth		
Neck		

Techniques	Data

Lungs

Heart

Abdomen

Musculoskeletal

20. What techniques did the nurse practitioner use to assess Paul's genitalia?

21. Describe the approach to examination of the genitalia in a 2-year-old male. (*Hint:* For more information on genitalia assessment, consult Chapter 7 in your textbook.)

LESSON 6

Health Promotion

 Reading Assignment: Perspectives of Pediatric Nursing (Chapter 1)
Family Influences on Child Health Promotion (Chapter 3)
Health Promotion of the Infant and Family (Chapter 10)
Health Promotion of the Toddler and Family (Chapter 12)

Patient: Paul Parker, Room 202

In this lesson the learner will review important aspects of toddler immunization needs. The learner will also describe important health promotion aspects appropriate for a toddler in relation to parent teaching for injury prevention.

CD-ROM Activity

For this lesson, you will again be working in the Well-Child Clinic (Floor 2). Click on the **Login Computer** in the Nurses' Station and sign in to work with Paul Parker. If you need to refamiliarize yourself with Paul's condition, review the Case Overview, as well as the Birth & Health History section of his Chart. Next, observe the Parent Interview with Paul's mother. Afterward, return to the Nurses' Station, click on **Anticipatory Guidance** and review these documents.

1. Which of the following is not among the top five types of injury among toddlers? (*Hint:* For more information on common types of toddler injuries, review Chapter 1 in your textbook.)
   a. Motor vehicle accident
   b. Drowning
   c. Choking/suffocation
   d. Firearm
   e. Burn

2. Describe five safety measures parents should be taught to decrease the risk for falls at home. Were these safety measures discussed with Paul's mother?

3. What temperature is considered safe for household water heaters?
   a. 125° F
   b. 120° F
   c. 90° F
   d. 95° F

4. Name at least three types of poisoning commonly experienced by toddlers, and explain why these poisonings usually occur.

5. Where are most of the toxic substances found in family households?
   a. Bathroom
   b. Kitchen
   c. Basement
   d. Bedroom

6. What instructions should be given to Paul's mother regarding the use of ipecac syrup if Paul were to ingest a noncorrosive toxic substance at home?

7. Several commonly used over-the-counter medications can cause serious or fatal consequences in children. Identify at least two of these substances, and describe what you would discuss with Paul's mother to prevent accidents.

8. Nursing caries is a dental concern for children. At what age is this usually found? When should Paul visit a dentist?

9. Many toddlers are afraid to go to the dentist. What can you discuss with Paul's mother to make the visit easier for him?

→ Return to Paul's Chart and click on **Immunization Record**. Review these records and refer to the Birth & Health History section of the Chart as needed to answer the following questions.

10. Review Paul's immunization status. Are his immunizations up to date? What immunizations are needed next, and when should they be administered?

11. What documentation is necessary when administering an immunization? What is documented in Paul's Chart?

12. Why did Paul receive the vaccine Prevnar?

13. Should Paul's mother be advised to give him low-fat milk or whole milk? Why?

14. Paul's mother is concerned about the amount of food Paul is eating. What is a general guide to appropriate serving sizes of food for toddlers?

15. Which of the following should Paul be doing by 2 years of age? Check all that apply.

    a. _____   Uses straw and cup
    b. _____   Uses fork correctly
    c. _____   Knows difference between finger and spoon foods
    d. _____   Uses adult patterns of chewing
    e. _____   Uses spoon

16. Which of the following are appropriate strategies to use during a time-out for a 2 year-old child? Check all that apply.

    a. _____   Select an area for time-out that is safe and convenient
    b. _____   Place the child in time-out for 10 minutes each time
    c. _____   Use a timer to record the time rather than a watch
    d. _____   Never implement time-out in a public place
    e. _____   Allow them to have a favorite toy with them

17. What advice can you give Paul's mother on using "consequences" for Paul at this age?

18. Describe some of the strategies to promote family relationships that should be discussed during the health visit.

LESSON 7

Growth and Development

👓 **Reading Assignment:** Health Promotion of the Preschooler and Family (Chapter 13)

Patient: Sherrie Bedonie, Room 204

This lesson will acquaint the learner with aspects of preschooler growth and development, as well as some of the major milestones of this age group. A review of the physical growth patterns during the first 4 years of life is also included.

💿 **CD-ROM Activity**

Go to the Well-Child Clinic on Floor 2 and sign in to work with Sherrie Bedonie. After hearing the Case Overview and reading the assignment, go to the Nurses' Station. Click on **Parent Interview** and pay particular attention to the Health Supervision segment. Finally, return to the Nurses' Station and open Sherrie's Chart. Click on **Developmental Surveillance** and review the section completed at 24 months of age.

1. When she was 24 months old, was Sherrie doing developmental tasks appropriate for her age?

2. What developmental tasks did Sherrie exhibit at 24 months?

3. Give three examples of appropriate toys that could have been discussed with Sherrie's parents to promote development at 24 months of age.

4. At what age should Sherrie have been doing each of the following?

_____	Transfers cubes from hand to hand	a. 4 months
_____	Sits with support	b. 24 months
_____	Drinks from cup	c. 7 months
_____	Rolls over	d. 12 months
_____	Listens to story	e. 16 months
_____	Can speak 15 to 20 words	f. 6 months
_____	Can use two-word phrases	g. 18 months

→ Return to the Developmental Surveillance section of Sherrie's Chart. Review her reports beginning at 6 months of age.

5. Is Sherrie progressing appropriately in relation to developmental milestones for her age? Give specific examples to support your answer.

6. The preschool period is characterized by refinement of gross and fine motor skills. Give examples of these types of skills demonstrated by Sherrie.

7. Which of the following tasks is/are appropriate to assess development of a 4-year-old? Check all that apply.

a. _____   Builds 10-block tower
b. _____   Hops on one foot
c. _____   Recognizes letters
d. _____   Knows address
e. _____   Throws ball overhand

Review the developmental assessment found in Sherrie's Chart.

8. Is Sherrie demonstrating appropriate tasks (as identified in question 7) for a child her age?

 9. Describe the preschool period according to Erikson. (*Hint:* For more information on the work of Erikson, read the section on development in Chapter 13 of your textbook.)

10. What does Erikson call this period?

11. How might you further assess Sherrie's sense of initiative? Develop three questions that could be used to assess this stage of her development.

 12. According to Piaget, in what phase of development is Sherrie presently? (*Hint:* Review Chapter 13 in your textbook for more information regarding Piaget.)

13. Describe this phase of development according to Piaget's cognitive theory.

14. Describe three activities that could be used to assess this phase of cognitive development.

➡ Return to Sherrie's Chart and review the Growth Charts section.

15. Calculate the percentiles for Sherrie's head circumference at the following ages:

    a. 12 months of age = _____%

    b. 18 months of age = _____%

    c. 24 months of age = _____%

16. What do your findings in question 15 tell you?

17. Assess Sherrie's height and weight during the first 24 months of life according to standard growth charts.

18. Plot Sherric's present weight and height on the growth chart below.

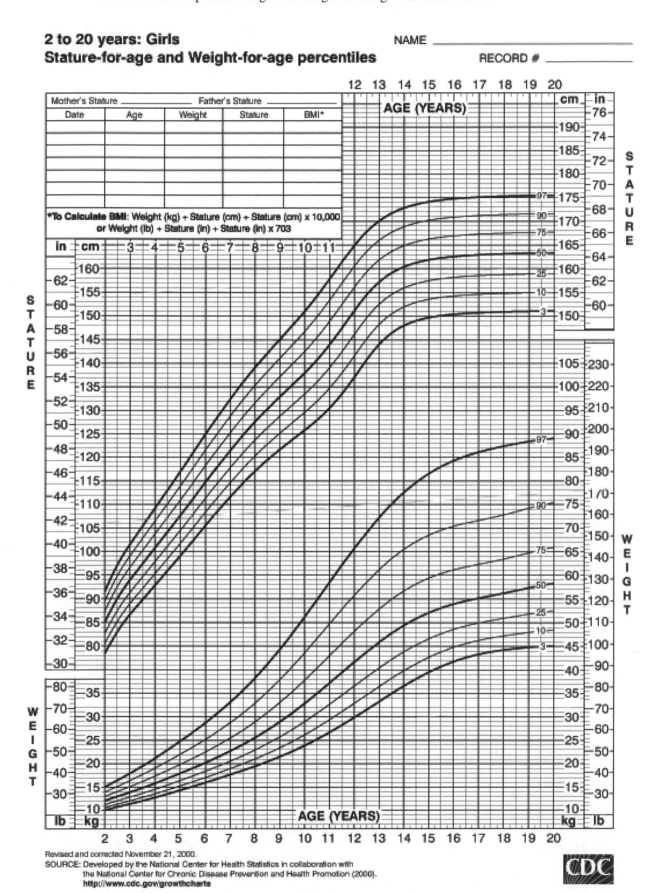

2 to 20 years: Girls
Stature-for-age and Weight-for-age percentiles

NAME _____

RECORD # _____

Mother's Stature _____ Father's Stature _____

Date	Age	Weight	Stature	BMI*

*To Calculate BMI: Weight (kg) ÷ Stature (cm) ÷ Stature (cm) x 10,000
or Weight (lb) ÷ Stature (in) ÷ Stature (in) x 703

Revised and corrected November 21, 2000.
SOURCE: Developed by the National Center for Health Statistics in collaboration with
the National Center for Chronic Disease Prevention and Health Promotion (2000).
http://www.cdc.gov/growthcharts

19. Explain why it is appropriate to evaluate weight and height over time in children.

20. What is the average weight and height for a 4-year-old girl?

Weight

Height

21. Approximately how much weight is gained per year on average during the preschool period?

22. Play during the preschool years is essential for promoting continued physical, social, and mental development. For each of these areas, identify three examples of play activities that promote development in the preschool child. (*Hint:* Consult the section on development in Chapter 13 of your textbook and review the growth and development assessment on the CD-ROM if you need assistance.)

Physical

Social

Mental

History and Physical Assessment

📖 **Reading Assignment:** Physical and Developmental Assessment of the Child (Chapter 7)
Health Problems of the Newborn and Family (Chapter 8)
Health Promotion of the Preschooler and Family (Chapter 13)
Impact of Cognitive or Sensory Impairment on the Child and Family (Chapter 19)

Patient: Sherrie Bedonie, Room 204

This lesson will acquaint the learner with aspects of the history and physical assessment of a 48-month-old well child. The learner will review techniques for performing a physical assessment of a child and what some of the important findings represent at this age. Assessment of vital signs and hearing and vision testing will all be examined. Anticipatory guidance issues will be presented as they relate to the child's status in the existing family structure.

💿 **CD-ROM Activity**

You will continue working with Sherrie Bedonie in the Well-Child Clinic. Access the Login Computer in the Nurses' Station on Floor 2 and select Sherrie as your patient. Then click on **Patient Records** and review the following sections of Sherrie's Chart: Birth & Health History, Well-Child Visits, Sick-Child Visits, Immunization Record, and Growth Charts.

1. What essential parts of the Birth & Health History section of the Chart should be reviewed with the mother of a 4-year-old well child?

2. Record Sherrie's weight, length, and head circumference at birth. Are these appropriate parameters for a newborn according to the Growth Charts section of the Chart?

3. What were Sherrie's Apgar and Ballard scores at the time of delivery? Describe the components of each test. (*Hint:* Review the information on newborn screening tools in Chapter 8 of your textbook.)

4. Do you have any concerns for Sherrie's future health, based on her family health history?

→ Return to Sherrie's Chart and review her examination records in the Hearing & Vision Screening section.

5. Records indicate that Sherrie passed the hearing screen at 20 dB at a frequency level of 4000 Hz. What is the representative sound at this level?

 6. If a child has mild to moderate hearing loss, at what decibel (dB) can he or she hear? What effect would this have on the child's hearing or speech? (*Hint:* Information regarding hearing impairment can be found in Chapters 7 and 19 of your textbook.)

7. What are some possible methods to promote cooperation of the preschool child during a hearing exam?

8. What were the results of Sherrie's vision screening examination? What conclusions can you draw from this finding?

 9. Name and describe three eye examination tests that are appropriate for preschool children. (*Hint:* Additional information on vision examination screenings may be found in Chapter 7 of your textbook.)

→ Return to the Nurses' Station and click on the **Physical Examination** button in the drop-down menu. Observe the nurse as she collects Sherrie's data during the physical assessment. After the exam is completed, return to the Nurses' Station, open Sherrie's Chart, and review the data in her Well-Child Visits section.

10. Are Sherrie's vital signs within normal limits for her age? If not, what parameters are abnormal in comparison with norms for a child her age? (*Hint:* Guidance on how to assess vital signs can be found in Chapter 7 in your textbook.)

11. Within what percentile range is Sherrie's blood pressure reading? What is the clinical significance of this finding?

12. Is there any cause for concern regarding Sherrie's vital signs? Explain. At what point would there be cause for concern?

13. By which method was Sherrie's temperature taken?
    a. Oral
    b. Rectal
    c. Tympanic
    d. Axillary

14. Describe what specific assessments the nurse conducted in each of the following areas of the physical examination. (*Hint:* If you need help, refer to textbook Chapter 7 for more about physical assessment techniques.)

Body Area	Assessment
Head	
Eyes	

Body Area	**Assessment**
Ears	
Mouth	
Neck	
Lungs	
Heart	
Abdomen	

15. What abnormal finding did you note as you observed the assessments listed in question 14?

16. What could be the possible cause of this abnormal finding, based on Sherrie's past health history?

➡️ Go to Sherrie's room and review the abdomen examination on the video of the physical assessment.

17. Describe the findings of the NP.

 18. Describe the sequence of the techniques used in the examination of the abdomen. Why is this sequence used? (*Hint:* Refer to Chapter 7 to learn more about the physical assessment of the abdomen.)

➡️ Review the heart assessment of the chest and back portion of Sherrie's physical examination.

19. What procedures were performed to complete the heart assessment?

20. What were the NP's findings from the heart assessment?

 21. Review the examination of the heart found in Chapter 7. At what location are the following sounds heard the loudest, and what causes the sound?

Sound	Location	Cause of the Sound
S_1		
S_2		

Health Promotion

Reading Assignment: Health Promotion of the Infant and Family (Chapter 10)
Health Promotion of the Toddler and Family (Chapter 12)
Health Promotion of the Preschooler and Family (Chapter 13)

Patient: Sherrie Bedonie, Room 204

In this lesson the learner will review important aspects of health promotion for the preschool child. The learner will also review the immunization needs of a preschooler and determine the major safety concerns. Anticipatory guidance issues will be presented as they relate to the preschool child.

CD-ROM Activity

Once again, you will work with 4-year-old Sherrie Bedonie in the Well-Child Clinic on Floor 2. After you have signed in, click on **Anticipatory Guidance** on the drop-down menu and review this session. Next, open and review Sherrie's Chart, paying particular attention to the Well-Child Visits and Sick-Child Visits sections.

1. How has Sherrie's prior nutritional status been assessed?

2. What nutritional approaches would allow you to further evaluate the nutritional intake of a preschool child? (*Hint:* For more information, read the section on nutrition in Chapter 13 of your textbook.)

Close Sherrie's Chart and click on **Physical Examination** on the drop-down menu. Once inside Room 204, observe Sherrie's physical examination.

3. Sherrie is a Navajo Indian. What questions might be helpful in determining whether there are any cultural practices that may influence her nutritional status?

 Access Sherrie's Chart and review her History & Physical.

4. Which of the following can be indications of poor nutritional status in children? (Check all correct answers.)

a. _____   Dull, dry hair
b. _____   Poor growth
c. _____   Delayed fusion of sutures
d. _____   Tissues at inner corners of mouth
e. _____   Poor skin turgor

 Leave Sherrie's room and return to the Nurses' Station. Click on **Patient Records** to open Sherrie's Chart. Click on **Well-Child Visits** and review the form from Sherrie's most recent visit. What medications is she presently taking?

5. If the fluoride concentration is 0.3 ppm in the public water supply where Sherrie lives, does she need fluoride supplementation? If yes, how much fluoride supplementation does she need? (*Hint:* Refer to Chapter 12 of your textbook for information on fluoride supplementation.)

Continue to review the Well-Child Visits section of Sherrie's Chart as needed to answer the following questions.

6. How was Sherrie's sleep status evaluated? What is her sleep status?

7. The preschool period is often a time of numerous sleep problems. Describe two common sleep problems experienced during this period and identify interventions to help the child and parents with these difficulties.

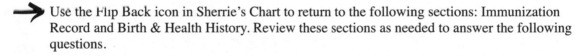 Use the Flip Back icon in Sherrie's Chart to return to the following sections: Immunization Record and Birth & Health History. Review these sections as needed to answer the following questions.

 8. Review Sherrie's immunization status. Are Sherrie's immunizations up to date? What immunizations will she need prior to starting a new school year? (*Hint:* To learn more about immunization schedules, go to Chapter 12 of your textbook.)

9. Why is IPV now recommended in the United States instead of OPV?

10. Water safety is a major concern for the preschool child; this was discussed with Sherrie's mother. Describe three important issues related to water safety that should be discussed with a parent of a preschooler. Circle the items related to water safety that were discussed with Sherrie's mother.

11. Based on Sherrie's age and weight, what safety measures are required when she rides in a motor vehicle?

12. What information should you provide to Sherrie's mother regarding the regulations for child car safety seats?

13. Which of the following statements are true regarding the use of car safety belts for a child Sherrie's age? Check all that are true.

    a. _____   Safety belts should be worn high on the hips.
    b. _____   Safety belts should fit across the abdominal area.
    c. _____   The child should sit up straight.
    d. _____   Shoulder belts should not cross the neck or face.

14. Describe the bicycle helmet that provides the best protection for a child Sherrie's age.

15. What safety questions should you ask Sherrie's mother regarding the presence of firearms in the home?

16. Which of the following age-related issues were discussed with Sherrie's mother? Check all that apply.

    _____   Expect nightmares at this age
    _____   Expect resistance to parental authority
    _____   Expect increased sexual curiosity
    _____   Remove drawstrings from clothing

17. Stranger safety is a big concern for preschoolers and their parents. Describe three interventions that should be discussed with Sherrie's mother to decrease the risk for abduction.

18. What specific issues is Sherrie's mother concerned about at this time?

19. How can school readiness be assessed in a preschool child?

20. The preschool period is a time of great sexual curiosity. What two rules govern answering sensitive questions about sex?

10

Signs and Symptoms of Childhood Leukemia

Reading Assignment: The Child with Hematologic or Immunologic Dysfunction (Chapter 26)

Patient: De Olp, Room 310

In this lesson, the student will learn to describe the signs and symptoms of childhood leukemia and bone marrow infiltration. The student will also learn to evaluate a complete blood cell count in the newly diagnosed child with leukemia.

CD-ROM Activity

Go to the Nurses' Station on the Pediatric Floor (Floor 3), locate the Login Computer, and sign in to work with De Olp at 0700. Watch the Case Overview and read through the Assignment. Then return to the Nurses' Station and open De's Chart. Review the following sections: History & Physical, Nursing History, and Laboratory Reports.

1. Based on your review of her history, what signs and symptoms did De present with that are suggestive of leukemia?
   a. Low-grade fever
   b. Fatigue and lethargy
   c. Pain in joints
   d. Gum bleeding
   e. All of the above

2. What findings from the physical examination are suggestive of leukemia?

3. Complete the following diagram on the signs and symptoms associated with bone marrow infiltration. First identify a symptom caused by a decrease in each of the listed cell counts. Then list three signs associated with each symptom. (*Hint:* To find out more about the signs and symptoms of leukemia, refer to Chapter 26 of your textbook.)

> ```
> ┌───────────────────────────┐
> │  Bone Marrow Infiltration │
> └───────────────────────────┘
> ```

	Decreased RBCs	Decreased WBCs	Decreased Platelets
Symptom	_____	_____	_____
Sign	_____	_____	_____
Sign	_____	_____	_____
Sign	_____	_____	_____

4. What was De's white blood cell (WBC) count at diagnosis? What is a normal range for WBC count for someone De's age? (*Hint:* If you need assistance, refer to Appendix E in your textbook.)

5. If a *decreased* WBC count can be a sign of leukemia, what might be an explanation for De's *elevated* WBC count?

6. Return to De's Chart and review the blood counts in the Laboratory Reports section. For each blood count listed below, record De's data for the 4 days specified.

Counts	Saturday PM	Sunday AM	Monday AM	Tuesday AM
WBC				
HgB				
Platelets				
Differential %				
Segs/Bands				
Lymphocytes				
Lymphoblasts				
Monocytes				
Eosinophils				
Basophils				

7. Based on a review of De's complete blood count (CBC) over the 4 days as recorded in question 6, what observation(s) can you make?

8. Why are these changes in De's CBC occurring? What might explain these findings?

9. Define *lymphoblasts* and explain why an overproduction of these cells would cause symptoms of leukemia. (*Hint:* For more information, see the discussion of leukemia in textbook Chapter 26.)

10. Did De present in any pain? If yes, what was the location of her pain?

11. How did leukemia cause pain in her knees and ankles? (*Hint:* If you need help, consult the section on leukemia in Chapter 26.)

12. In addition to the CBC findings, what other physical findings in De's case could be attributed to leukemia?

13. What causes swelling of the lymph nodes in patients with leukemia?

Treatment and Procedures

Reading Assignment: Family-Centered Care of the Child During Illness and
Hospitalization (Chapter 21)
Pediatric Variations of Nursing Interventions (Chapter 22)
The Child with Hematologic or Immunologic Dysfunction
(Chapter 26)

Patient: De Olp, Room 310

In this lesson, the learner will describe the diagnosis of leukemia and review the types of
chemotherapeutic treatments. The learner will also discuss the preparations prior to performing
invasive procedures.

CD-ROM Activity

In this lesson you will continue working with De Olp, so go to the Nurses' Station on the Pediatric Floor (Floor 3) and sign in to work with her at 1100. Review the Case Overview and the
Assignment. From the Nurses' Station, open De's Chart and review these sections: History &
Physical, Laboratory Reports, X-Rays & Diagnostics, Medication Records, and Nursing History.

1. How was De's diagnosis of leukemia confirmed? Describe the finding.

2. What could possibly explain the decrease in production of formed elements of the blood?

3. Review the cerebral spinal fluid analysis in the X-Rays & Diagnostics section of De's Chart. Why was it important to obtain a CSF analysis from De at the time of the diagnosis of leukemia?

4. What chemotherapy agent was administered to De by lumbar puncture? What dose was given?

 5. What is the most likely explanation for the administration of methotrexate? (*Hint:* For more information on the administration of methotrexate in patients with leukemia, refer to Chapter 26 in your textbook.)

→ Return to De's Chart and review the findings recorded in the Progress Notes section.

6. Proper preparation for invasive painful procedures in children is essential. How was De taught about these procedures? Is there anything else that you would have done or anything you would have done differently in teaching De? (*Hint:* For more information on preparation for procedures, review Chapter 22 of your textbook.)

7. Describe at least three guidelines that are helpful in preparing children for invasive procedures.

8. List at least four words or phrases to avoid when discussing De's treatment and procedures with her. For each word or phrase you identify, suggest a substitution.

Word/Phrase to Avoid	Suggested Substitution

➡ Again, return to De's Chart. This time, review Physician Orders and Medication Records.

9. Below, list all the medications De is receiving for her leukemia (including doses). Also describe how each medication is being administered.

Medication and Dose	How Medication Is Being Administered

10. Describe the major side effects associated with the use of vincristine (Oncovin).
(*Hint:* Review the chemotherapy table in Chapter 26 of your textbook.).

11. Describe the major side effects associated with the use of dexamethasone (Decadrol).

Potential Complications of Childhood Leukemia

📖 **Reading Assignment:** The Child with Gastrointestinal Dysfunction (Chapter 24)
The Child with Hematologic or Immunologic Dysfunction (Chapter 26)

Patient: De Olp, Room 310

In this lesson, the learner will identify the potential complications associated with the treatment for childhood leukemia. The learner will determine the daily fluid requirements of a child with leukemia and review the laboratory studies monitored during treatment. Nursing interventions that may prevent possible complications associated with the treatment of leukemia will also be described.

💿 **CD-ROM Activity**

In the Nurses' Station on the Pediatric Floor, go to the Login Computer and sign in to work with De Olp at 1100. After watching the Case Overview, click on the **Assignment** button and review the preceptor's summary and your assigned task. Then return to the Nurses' Station, open De's Chart, and read the Progress Notes.

1. Describe the events that took place on Tuesday morning that represent potential complications for De.

Access De's EPR (Electronic Patient Record) and click on **Input & Output**.

2. Review De's intake and output status from Monday at 2000 until Tuesday at 1000 (12 hours) and complete the following table.

	Monday	Tuesday		
	2000	0700	1000	Total
Intake				
Output				
Intake Minus Output				

 3. De weighs 18 kg. Calculate her daily maintenance IV fluid requirements. (*Hint:* To review maintenance fluids, refer to Chapter 24 in your textbook.)

4. De's IV rate is 95 mL/hour. Based on her body surface area or M^2, what is her fluid rate?

5. Why are De's fluids infusing at a rate greater than the recommended daily maintenance rate?

 Return to De's Chart and click on **Laboratory Reports**.

 6. For each lab test listed below, record De's results and the normal range for that test. Circle any of De's lab values that are abnormal. (*Hint:* Normal laboratory ranges can be found in Appendix E in your textbook).

Lab Test	De's Results Tuesday AM	Normal Range
Sodium		
Potassium		
Chloride		
CO^2		
Glucose		
BUN		
Creatinine		
Calcium		
Magnesium		
Phosphorus		
Uric Acid		

7. What are some possible reasons for De's weight gain and edema?

 8. What laboratory tests are ordered for every 12 hours in a child with leukemia? Why are they ordered at these intervals? (*Hint:* Review the leukemia section in textbook Chapter 26.)

→ Return to the Nurses' Station and click on the **Login Computer**. A Warning screen will appear informing you that you are already logged in for a patient. Click on **Supervisor's Computer** and then on **Nurses' Station**. This will allow you to sign out for this time period. Now, click again on the **Login Computer** and sign in to work with De Olp at 1300. After watching the Case Overview and reading the Assignment, return to the Nurses' Station and do the following:

- Open De's Chart and review the Physician Orders and Progress Notes. When you are finished, click on **Nurses' Station** to close the Chart.
- Access and review De's Medication Administration Record (MAR) by clicking on the notebook in the Nurses' Station or by using the drop-down menu.
- Close the MAR and open De's EPR. Click on **Respiratory** and review the data summary.

9. Based on De's data in the EPR, what respiratory findings changed between Tuesday 1230 and Tuesday 1300?

10. According to the Physician Orders in De's Chart, what concerns led to the ordering of a chest x-ray?

11. Use the space below to answer these questions: What medication was administered to De on Tuesday morning? What dose was given? What route of administration was used? Why was this drug administered?

Drug	Dose	Route	Reason for Administration

 12. Describe at least three nursing observations necessary in preventing fluid abnormalities in a patient with leukemia. (*Hint:* Review fluid overload in Chapter 22 of your textbook.)

13

Psychosocial Aspects of Care

👓 **Reading Assignment:** Impact of Chronic Illness, Disability, or Death on the Child and Family (Chapter 18)
Family-Centered Care of the Child During Illness and Hospitalization (Chapter 21)
The Child with Hematologic or Immunologic Dysfunction (Chapter 26)

Patient: De Olp, Room 310

In this lesson, the learner will describe the important aspects of a psychosocial assessment and review the emotions associated with a recent diagnosis of childhood cancer. The learner will also learn to evaluate nursing interventions that promote independence and control for a school-age child and describe the nursing actions that promote understanding of the illness and treatment.

💿 **CD-ROM Activity**

Once again, you will work with De Olp, this time during the 1100–1229 period of care. Sign in for this patient and period of care on the Login Computer on Floor 3. Before you complete the following CD-ROM activities, read through all questions in this lesson to guide your review. Take notes as you review De's records.

- Open De's Chart and review the History & Physical and Nursing History, paying particular attention to the assessment of the family's and De's support network.

1. After reviewing assessments in the History & Physical provided by the ED staff and the physician, describe De's psychosocial environment.

2. Describe De's family support.

3. Describe the assessment of De's school performance. (*Hint:* Return to the Nursing History in her Chart, if necessary.)

→ Visit De in her room (Room 310) and click on the **Behavior** button in the lower left corner, below the body model. One at a time, select the following buttons and review: Signs of Distress, Needs, and Support. Observe the nurse as she collects data regarding De's behavior.

4. Based on your review of De's Chart, describe the emotions that she is feeling.

5. Based on De's developmental level (school-age child), what issues may be most difficult for her as she faces her diagnosis? (*Hint:* For information on the impact of illness on the school-age child, refer to Chapter 18 in your textbook. Stressors of hospitalization can be found in Chapter 22.)

6. What nursing actions can facilitate De's needs and promote continued development during this time? (*Hint:* To find out more about helping pediatric patients minimize their loss of control, refer to that discussion in Chapter 21 in your textbook.)

7. A newly diagnosed child with cancer faces a great deal of uncertainty and fear related to the diagnosis. Describe at least three nursing interventions that will help De face her fears. (*Hint:* Information on nursing care of the child with cancer can be found in Chapter 26 of your textbook.)

 8. Describe at least three factors that may influence De's father's reaction to his daughter's illness. (*Hint:* These factors can be found in the family section of textbook Chapter 18.)

9. Helping the family members communicate their needs for information about De's diagnosis is an important nursing intervention. Describe at least three guidelines that would facilitate the family's ability to gain information about the diagnosis and treatment.

10. List three questions that could be used to assess the family's ability to cope with the new diagnosis. (*Hint:* Information about assessment questions can be found in Chapter 26 in your textbook.)

 11. When working with families of children with a chronic illness it is important to develop successful parent-professional partnerships. Identify ways to promote development of these relationships. (*Hint:* For more on parent-professional relationships, review Chapter 18 of your textbook.)

Kaylie Sern

Culture and the Community

Reading Assignment: Perspectives of Pediatric Nursing (Chapter 1)
Family Influences on Child Health Promotion (Chapter 3)
Social, Cultural, and Religious Influences on Child Health
Promotion (Chapter 4)
Developmental Influences on Child Health Promotion
(Chapter 5)
Communication and Health Assessment of the Child and Family
(Chapter 6)
Pediatric Variations of Nursing Interventions (Chapter 22)

Patient: Kaylie Sern, Room 304

This lesson will focus on aspects of nursing care related to the patient's culture and community
with emphasis on her role within the foster family and their community.

 CD-ROM Activity

Go to the Nurses' Station on the Pediatric Floor (Floor 3) and locate the Login Computer. Sign
in to work with Kaylie Sern at 0700 and review the Case Overview and your Assignment.
Return to the Nurses' Station, open Kaylie's Chart, and review her Nursing History.

Writing Activity

1. What is the term for the type of family in which Kaylie lives?

2. Based on the data in the Nursing Admissions Pediatric Patient Profile, list four family
   strengths of Kaylie's family.

3. Based on the data in the Nursing Admissions Profile, does Kaylie appear to be integrated into this family as an integral family member? Provide two specific examples to substantiate your response.

➤ Open the Kardex and review Kaylie's Patient Care Plan. Then return to her Chart and read the History & Physical and Physician Orders. Now return to the Nurses' Station, click **Patient Care** from the drop-down menu, and select **Data Collection**. Once inside Kaylie's room, observe the nurse as she conducts a complete physical examination.

4. Briefly describe examples of the pediatric nurse's role in relation to Kaylie's care in the hospital.

5. Based on the available data in Kaylie's Chart, describe for each of the following areas any special cultural factors that need to be considered and incorporated into Kaylie's care.

   a. Family structure/function

   b. Health beliefs

c. Religious beliefs

d. Food customs

6. According to Erikson's theory of personality development, Kaylie is in what psychosocial stage of development? (*Hint:* For more information on psychosocial development, refer to Chapter 5 in your textbook.)

7. Briefly describe three characteristics of the developmental stage you identified in question 6.

8. According to Piaget's theory of cognitive development, Kaylie is in the preoperational stage of intellectual development. How does knowledge of the characteristics of this stage influence your plan of care for Kaylie in the hospital setting? (*Hint:* For more information on cognitive development, refer to Chapter 5 in your textbook.)

9. Kaylie has an IV in her left hand. Describe her behavior during the physical assessment in relation to the IV. Does the IV appear to affect her body image? What other evidence does she display during her examination that is strongly representative of a child her age? (*Hint:* To learn more about preventing or minimizing bodily injury, refer to Chapter 21 in your textbook; to learn about the development of body image, consult Chapter 13.)

→ Return to the Nurses' Station and open Kaylie's Chart. Click on **Nursing History** and review the Nursing Admissions Pediatric Patient Profile. Then close the Chart, open the Kardex, and review Kaylie's Patient Care Plan.

10. Describe three play activities that would be appropriate for Kaylie to engage in. For each example, provide a brief rationale for the appropriateness of the activity.

Physical Assessment

📖 **Reading Assignment:** Communication and Health Assessment of the Child and Family (Chapter 6)
Physical and Developmental Assessment of the Child (Chapter 7)
The Child with Respiratory Dysfunction (Chapter 23)
The Child with Gastrointestinal Dysfunction (Chapter 24)

Patient: Kaylie Sern, Room 304

In this lesson, important aspects of the physical examination of a 3-year-old child with dehydration and otitis media will be covered. Physical examination data will be linked to the child's hydration status and nursing measures aimed at improving hydration status and maintaining appropriate skin integrity.

💿 **CD-ROM Activity**

Begin this exercise by going to the Nurses' Station on the Pediatric Floor (Floor 3). Locate the Login Computer and sign in to work with Kaylie Sern at 0700. After watching the Case Overview and reviewing the Assignment, return to the Nurses' Station and open Kaylie's Chart. Review her History & Physical. Then close the Chart and go to visit Kaylie in her room. Observe the nurse as she conducts a complete physical examination. Be sure to take notes about the nurse's findings.

1. How does Kaylie react as the nurse takes her vital signs and performs a physical assessment? What is Kaylie's reaction to these interventions? Based on your knowledge of her developmental stage, what specific action(s) could the nurse take to decrease Kaylie's anxiety and discomfort while obtaining vital signs and performing a head-to-toe physical examination?

2. How is Kaylie described in the History & Physical with respect to her level of activity and consciousness? What is the significance of these findings?

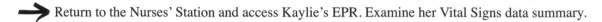 Return to the Nurses' Station and access Kaylie's EPR. Examine her Vital Signs data summary.

3. Kaylie's vital signs are recorded by the nurse on the EPR. What was her initial heart rate and temperature at 0600?

 4. Listed below are findings noted in Kaylie's History & Physical. Circle all of the findings that are directly related to dehydration. (*Hint:* To learn more about the significance of clinical findings in relation to dehydration, refer to textbook Chapter 24.)

Skin: hot to touch, flushed

Respirations: nonlabored, 30 per minute

Neck: supple

Eyes: sunken, no tears

Oral mucosa: dry

Lips: dry

Bowel sounds: present in all four quadrants

Last urine output: 3:00 p.m. of previous day

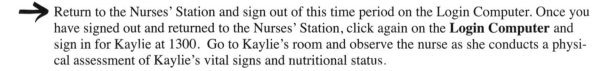 Return to the Nurses' Station and sign out of this time period on the Login Computer. Once you have signed out and returned to the Nurses' Station, click again on the **Login Computer** and sign in for Kaylie at 1300. Go to Kaylie's room and observe the nurse as she conducts a physical assessment of Kaylie's vital signs and nutritional status.

5. Kaylie's nurse performs a physical assessment at 1300. What does the nurse tell the mother about Kaylie's hydration status at this time?

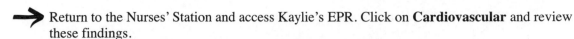

Return to the Nurses' Station and access Kaylie's EPR. Click on **Cardiovascular** and review these findings.

6. Based on the cardiovascular data in Kaylie's EPR, chart below how her skin, color, and turgor change during the following Tuesday time periods.

	0600	0900	1100	1300
Skin				
Color				
Turgor				

7. What specific request does Kaylie's nurse make of the mother when Kaylie indicates she needs to void. What is the significance of the nurse's request in relation to Kaylie's illness?

Return to the Nurses' Station and again access Kaylie's Chart. Review her Laboratory Reports.

8. What was the specific gravity of Kaylie's urine on Tuesday at 1030? What is the significance of this finding?

Close the Chart and return to Kaylie's room. Review her physical examination as needed to answer questions 13 through 20.

9. During Kaylie's physical examination at 1300, how is her mental status and activity level described? (*Hint:* Return to the videos for Initial Observations, Vital Signs, Head & Neck, and Behavior if needed.)

10. How is Kaylie's abdomen and bowel function evaluated by the nurse?

11. How does the nurse evaluate the condition of Kaylie's IV site and the functioning of the IV delivery equipment?

12. List three physical findings for which the nurse must be vigilant because they are indicative of complications of intravenous therapy in children. (*Hint:* To review parenteral fluid therapy, refer to Chapter 32 of your textbook.)

13. Describe how the nurse evaluates Kaylie's pulmonary and respiratory status.

14. Of the following findings, which is the most important determinant of hydration status in a young child?
    a. Skin turgor
    b. Body weight
    c. Level of consciousness
    d. Child's statement that she is thirsty

15. What does PERRLA mean? What are the results of Kaylie's EENT examination at 1300 on Tuesday? (*Hint:* If you need help, refer to Chapter 7 in your textbook.)

16. How does the nurse evaluate musculoskeletal status in Kaylie's upper and lower extremities?

Care of the Hospitalized Child

👓 **Reading Assignment:** Family-Centered Care of the Child During Illness and
Hospitalization (Chapter 21)
Pediatric Variations of Nursing Interventions (Chapter 22)

Patient: Kaylie Sern, Room 304

This lesson will introduce the learner to the general care of the preschool child who is hospitalized with an acute illness. The impact of hospitalization upon the child and the family unit will be a focus of the lesson, with attention also given to the child's acute illness and nursing care in acute care.

 CD-ROM Activity

In this lesson, you will continue working with Kaylie Sern. Go to the Nurses' Station on the Pediatric Floor and sign in to work with her at 1300. After watching the Case Overview and reviewing your Assignment, go into Kaylie's room and watch the Initial Observations and Behavior video segments. Return to the Nurses' Station and access Kaylie's Chart. Look over her History & Physical and Nursing History. As you review these sections, consider Kaylie's age, her family situation, and the fact that this is her first hospitalization.

✒ **Writing Activity**

1. Describe methods you observed on the video to minimize the trauma of hospitalization for Kaylie's family. Identify any methods noted in the Chart that might accomplish the same goal.

2. What additional methods may be implemented by the nursing staff to minimize the trauma of hospitalization for Kaylie? (*Hint:* If you need help, refer to Chapter 21 in your textbook for information on preventing or minimizing separation.)

→ Return to the Nurses' Station and enter Kaylie's room. Observe the nurse as she conducts a physical examination.

3. Identify one treatment modality that may represent a threat to Kaylie's body image and describe an appropriate way to minimize this perceived threat. Identify something you saw on the video in Kaylie's hospital room or her environment that could easily be altered or otherwise used to minimize her distress without compromising her treatment. (*Hint:* To learn ways to help minimize a pediatric patient's loss of control, consult textbook Chapter 21.)

4. What information did you read about Kaylie in her Chart that would help the nurse plan activities for her while hospitalized? (*Hint:* Return to the Nursing Admissions Pediatric Profile in the Nursing History section of Kaylie's Chart for help.)

5. Kaylie's mother, Shannon, expresses concern that Kaylie may wet the bed at night since it occurred during a previous illness. How is this concern best answered from a developmental perspective?

6. What activity do all children engage in that can be used in the hospital setting to decrease anxiety and minimize the trauma of hospitalization?

7. Play is an important part of a child's life. Identify an example of play that you saw Kaylie involved in during one of the videos during the course of her hospitalization.

→ Kaylie's mother calls the front desk and says she believes Kaylie is in pain. Go to the Chart and review the Physician Orders for Kaylie. Then return to the Nurses' Station, open Kaylie's MAR, and review those records.

8. If it is presently 1300, how long has it been since Kaylie last received a pain medication?

→ Return to the Nurses' Station and access the EPR. Click on **Vital Signs** and review Kaylie's pain ratings.

9. Record Kaylie's pain ratings for the times listed below.

Tuesday 0715   **Tuesday 0900**   **Tuesday 1000**

10. Kaylie's mother indicates that her daughter is no longer nauseated. What pain medication would you administer? By what route? Chart this medication on the sample MAR below as you would on Kaylie's MAR for Tuesday at 1300.

Patient:	MRN:	Room:	Date:

Medication Administration Record			
Medication	2300–0700	0700–1500	1500–2300

11. What antibiotic is Kaylie receiving, and at what time is the next antibiotic dose due according to the current MAR? (*Hint:* It is currently 1100 on Tuesday).

12. The antibiotic is available in a concentration of 250 mg/5 ml. The proper dose to administer

    is _____ ml.

13. Based on Kaylie's age, what would be the *best* way to administer the suspension (i.e., with a syringe, medication cup, or other method)? (*Hint:* If you need help, refer to the administration of medication section in textbook Chapter 22.)

14. Before discharge, the physician orders acetaminophen and ibuprofen for ear pain. Ibuprofen is administered every 6 hours in a dose of 10 mg/kg for pain and fever. Children's Motrin is available in suspension as 100 mg/5 ml.

    a. Calculate Kaylie's dosage of ibuprofen in milligrams, based on her weight of 15 kilograms.

    b. Calculate the number of milliliters of Children's Motrin you will administer to Kaylie.

→ Return to Kaylie's Chart and review the Physician Orders for items related to possible complications in Kaylie's case.

15. What order did you find related to a potential complication that Kaylie may experience as a result of her illness and for which the nurse must be vigilant? (*Hint:* Refer to textbook Chapter 22 for information on controlling elevated temperatures. See Chapter 28 to learn more about febrile seizures.)

16. What nursing measures must be taken to prevent Kaylie from harming herself in the event of febrile seizures?

 17. What nonpharmacologic activity is noted in Kaylie's History & Physical with respect to her parents' attempts to control her fever? Is this an appropriate treatment? In addition to the administration of an antipyretic, what anticipatory guidance might be given regarding methods to reduce body temperature at home? (*Hint:* For more on controlling elevated temperatures, refer to Chapter 22 in your textbook.)

Imbalance of Body Fluids

 Reading Assignment: Family-Centered Care of the Child During Illness and
Hospitalization (Chapter 21)
Pediatric Variations of Nursing Interventions (Chapter 22)

Patient: Kaylie Sern, Room 304

Objectives

This lesson deals with the child with an imbalance of fluid and electrolytes in the acute care
setting. The lesson will cover aspects of nursing care related to fluid replacement and monitoring of a child's fluid status in acute care.

CD-ROM Activity

Once again, you will care for Kaylie Sern on the Pediatric Floor (Floor 3). Locate the Login
Computer in the Nurses' Station and sign in to work with her at 0700. From the Nurses' Station,
open Kaylie's Chart and review her History & Physical and the Physician Orders. While reviewing these records, look for items related to her hydration status (fluid intake and output).

Writing Activity

1. What are Kaylie's primary medical diagnoses according to the Physician Orders? What procedures or treatments were performed in the ED for these diagnoses?

 2. What three factors lead to Kaylie's deteriorating hydration status? (*Hint:* Consult Chapter
   24 in your textbook for information on disturbances of fluid and electrolyte balance.)

137

3. What factors cause children Kaylie's age and size to become dehydrated more rapidly than adolescents or adults? (*Hint:* Refer to Chapter 28 in your textbook.)

4. What physical signs does Kaylie have that indicate a dehydration status?

5. Given Kaylie's hydration status and accompanying illness on Tuesday morning (0700), list three possible nursing diagnoses.

→ Return to Kaylie's Chart and click on **Laboratory Reports**.

6. Listed below are the results of Kaylie's 0600 urinalysis. Circle any abnormal finding(s) that is/are commonly seen in dehydration.

Glucose:	negative
Ketones:	negative
Spec. Gravity:	1.035
Blood:	negative
pH:	7.0
Protein:	negative
Nitrite:	negative
Leukocytes:	negative
WBC:	negative
Bacteria:	negative

7. Below, record Kaylie's electrolyte values from her 0615 chemistry profile in the Laboratory Reports section of her Chart. Then provide the normal range of values for each electrolyte in a child of Kaylie's age. Next, circle the two critically important electrolytes that should be monitored in a child with dehydration. Finally, place an asterisk next to any other electrolyte values that are out of the normal range. (*Hint:* Normal ranges of lab values can be found in Appendix D of your textbook.)

Electrolytes (Serum)	Kaylie's Values	Normal Ranges
Glucose		
Sodium		
Potassium		
Chloride		
CO_2		
Creatinine		
BUN		

8. Kaylie's parents express concern that she is not receiving any solid foods and that she will continue to lose weight. How should you counsel them regarding this concern?

➡ Return to the Nurses' Station and open and review Kaylie's MAR. Then return to Kaylie's Chart and review the Physician Orders. Watch specifically for diet instructions.

9. What medication does Kaylie's physician order to control nausea and vomiting?

10. What does the physician order related to oral rehydration for Kaylie? What is the rationale for these instructions? (*Hint:* for more information on diarrhea-therapeutic management, refer to Chapter 24 in your textbook.)

You have completed your CD-ROM activities for the current period. Return to the Nurses' Station and sign out on the Login Computer. Now sign in for Kaylie at 1300. After watching the Case Overview and reading the Assignment, go to Kaylie's room and observe the nurse as she collects data related to the following assessment areas: Vital Signs, Head and Neck, Upper Extremities, and Nutrition. When you have finished, return to the Nurses' Station and open Kaylie's Chart. This time, review the Progress Notes for Tuesday at 1000 and 1200.

11. Based on the videos you observed and your review of the Progress Notes, what specific methods does the nurse use to assess Kaylie's hydration status?

12. What does the nurse document in the 1300 Progress Notes that signals Kaylie's improving hydration status?

13. List four physical findings obtained during the 1300 physical examination that are indicative of improving hydration status.

14. Kaylie's parents express concern regarding her increased activity level and the IV in her left hand. They are worried she should remain in bed to avoid pulling out the IV. What is the best response to their concerns?

15. What important assessment data should be recorded regarding the IV site? Record these data on the sample Progress Note below as you would if making an official entry into the Chart.

Canyon View Regional Medical Center 1500 Sandstone Drive Canyon View, Arizona	MRN: Patient: Sex: Age: Room: Physician:

Progress Notes

Day	Time	Notes	Physician or Nurse

LESSON 18

Physical Assessment

 Reading Assignment: Physical and Developmental Assessment of the Child
(Chapter 7)

Patient: Jason Baker, Room 306

This lesson introduces the learner to a 14-year-old trauma victim, Jason Baker. In this lesson the learner will explore aspects of a health history and physical assessment as they relate to an adolescent who is hospitalized. The learner will review important considerations as they relate to the client's developmental stage, age, and acute care status.

 CD-ROM Activity

Begin this lesson by going to the Nurses' Station on the Surgery Floor (Floor 4). Locate the Login computer and sign in to work with Jason Baker in the PACU at 0930. After watching the Case Overview and reading the Preceptor Notes in the Assignment, return to the Nurses' Station and access Jason's Chart. Review his History & Physical, looking for items related to Jason's physical findings.

Writing Activity

1. What is the purpose of obtaining a health history on Jason at this time?

→ Visit Jason's room and observe the nurse's assessment of his head and neck.

2. According to the preadmission History & Physical, Jason has PERRLA. What is PERRLA? How did the nurse assess for PERRLA on the video?

➡ Now conduct an assessment of Jason's upper extremities.

3. What are the physical findings regarding Jason's upper extremity peripheral pulses? On the diagram below, mark with an X the location of four pulses that can be tested in an adolescent of Jason's age. Identify each pulse by name next to its location.

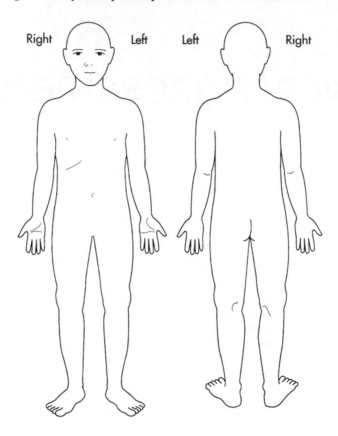

Right   Left   Left   Right

Now observe the nurse as she performs Jason's chest and back assessment. Also review the respiratory assessment performed by the nurse.

4. On the diagram below, mark each appropriate area of lung auscultation with an X.

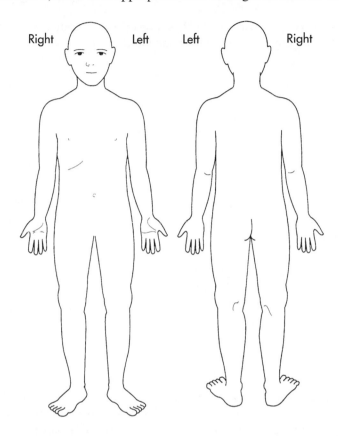

5. What is the clinical significance of performing a baseline preoperative pulmonary assessment and a comprehensive postoperative pulmonary assessment in a patient who undergoes general anesthesia?

 Still in Jason's room, click on **Vital Signs** and watch as the nurse collects a full set of vital signs data.

 6. Describe how the nurse measures Jason's oxygen saturation. What is his oxygen saturation reading, and what is the clinical significance of this finding? (*Hint:* Refer to Chapter 22 in your textbook for information on monitoring oxygen therapy.)

7. Based on your observation of Jason's respiratory pattern on the video (as reflected by the breathing body model), Jason's respirations are primarily:
   a. abdominal.
   b. diaphragmatic.

8. Would you characterize the chest movement in Jason's respiratory pattern as regular or irregular? Give specific information to substantiate your answer.

 9. Describe the expected location of the PMI (point of maximal impulse) during an auscultation of Jason's heart sounds. (*Hint:* Refer to Chapter 7 in your textbook if you need assistance.)

→ Return to the Nurses' Station and sign out for this period of care. Then take the elevator to the Pediatric Floor (Floor 3). Click on the **Nurses' Station** to enter the floor. Locate the Login Computer and sign in to work with Jason at 1100. Visit Jason's room and observe the nurse collect his vital signs data.

10. What is Jason's heart rate following transfer to his room? What is the normal heart rate range for an adolescent? (*Hint:* Normal heart ranges can be found on the inside back cover of your textbook.)

→ Still in Jason's room, observe as the nurse assesses Jason's wound condition and examines his lower extremities.

11. Describe the condition of Jason's right leg postoperatively. Note the presence of any significant physical findings.

12. Because Jason had orthopedic surgery on a limb, it is particularly important to examine what factors in regard to potential complications? Describe how the nurse examines Jason's lower extremities with respect to neurologic and muscular function.

13. How does the nurse evaluate Jason's genitourinary and bowel function?

14. Considering the fact that Jason is 14 years old, what is the most appropriate approach to the physical assessment of his genitourinary system?

15. Describe the location of Jason's peripheral intravenous infusion. What assessments should be made regarding his IV? Document your assessment of the infusion and site on the sample Progress Note below.

Canyon View Regional Medical Center 1500 Sandstone Drive Canyon View, Arizona	MRN: Patient: Sex: Age: Room: Physician:

Progress Notes

Day	Time	Notes	Physician or Nurse

Care of the Hospitalized Adolescent

✐ **Reading Assignment:** Health Promotion of the Adolescent and Family (Chapter 16)
Family-Centered Care of the Child During Illness and
Hospitalization (Chapter 21)
Pediatric Variations of Nursing Interventions (Chapter 22)
The Child with Musculoskeletal or Articular Dysfunction
(Chapter 31)

Patient: Jason Baker, Room 306

In this lesson the learner will work with an adolescent in the acute care setting for surgery and rehabilitation of a broken leg. Adolescence is a period of many developmental changes and challenges; restorative health care is an important focus of this lesson. The learner will also learn to work with health problems experienced by the adolescent client and devise appropriate pain management care for this client.

💿 **CD-ROM Activity**

Go to the Nurses' Station on the Surgery Floor (Floor 4), click on the **Login Computer**, and sign in to work with Jason Baker. Watch his Case Overview and read the Preceptor Note in his Assignment. Next, access his Chart and review the following sections: History & Physical, Nursing History, Operative Reports, and Physician Orders.

1. How does the physician order Jason's leg to be positioned? What is the purpose of placing his leg in this position?

→ Visit Jason in the Preoperative Care Bay. Click on **Initial Observations** and watch the video.

2. During preoperative care, what does the nurse ask Jason to do? What is the purpose in carrying out this intervention?

→ Go to the Nurses' Station and sign out for this period of care. Then return to the Login (Supervisor's) Computer and sign in to see Jason in the PACU at 0930. Access and review his Medication Administration Record (MAR). Then open his Chart and examine his Operative Reports.

3. What medication does Jason receive at 0725 prior to surgery? Identify the rationale for administering this medication to a patient in Jason's condition.

4. Describe the pain scale that is used to monitor Jason's leg pain. Is this an appropriate tool to use for an adolescent? What data support your answer? (*Hint:* For more on pain management, consult Chapter 21 in your textbook.)

5. What other data might be used to identify pain perception in an adolescent?

→ Still in Jason's Chart, click on **Physician Orders** and **Operative Reports**, reviewing each section.

6. Identify the medication(s) ordered for Jason's leg pain.

7. What are potential side effects for the medication Jason is receiving for pain?

8. Identify the potential side effect of this drug for which the PACU and pediatric nurses caring for Jason must be especially vigilant.

9. Define *equianalgesia* in terms related to Jason's pain status after surgery.

10. A morphine sulfate vial is labeled as follows: "Morphine sulfate 4 mg/ml." On the correct syringe below, indicate with an arrow how many milliliter of morphine should be drawn up for a dose of 3 mg. Shade the correct dosage on the syringe.

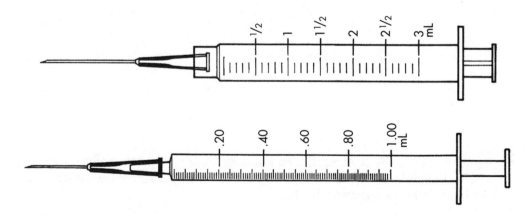

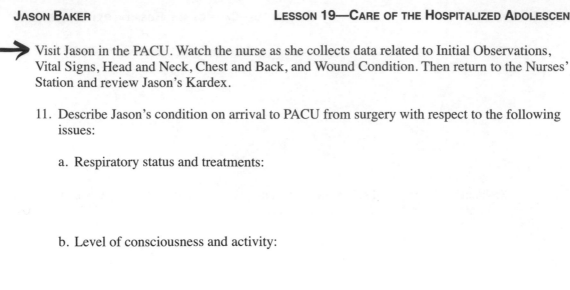

→ Visit Jason in the PACU. Watch the nurse as she collects data related to Initial Observations, Vital Signs, Head and Neck, Chest and Back, and Wound Condition. Then return to the Nurses' Station and review Jason's Kardex.

11. Describe Jason's condition on arrival to PACU from surgery with respect to the following issues:

   a. Respiratory status and treatments:

   b. Level of consciousness and activity:

   c. Pain sensation:

   d. Operative site:

→ Access Jason's Electronic Patient Record (EPR) and review his vital signs summary.

12. What were Jason's vital signs on arrival in the PACU? Compare these to baseline vitals taken at 0630. Are these vital signs within normal range for an adolescent, or is there need to contact the physician? Explain your answer.

→ Return to the Nurses' Station, click on **Planning Care** from the drop-down menu, and select **Setting Priorities**. Examine some of the possible nursing diagnoses and review the outcomes and interventions associated with them.

13. List two possible nursing diagnoses for Jason in the immediate postoperative period.

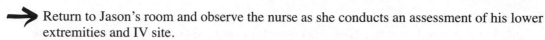 Return to Jason's room and observe the nurse as she conducts an assessment of his lower extremities and IV site.

14. Identify operative site assessments made by the nurse in PACU. List three critical assessments that reflect adequate vascular and neurologic function of the operated extremity.

15. What assessments does the PACU nurse make in regard to Jason's IV site, the equipment in his room, and the fluids infusing?

➡ Access Jason's Chart and click on **Operative Records**. Review the PACU discharge record on p. 12 of this section.

16. What oral intake did Jason have in PACU?

17. What is the rationale for oral intake limitations during the immediate postoperative period?

18. What specific physical assessment criteria would be used to advance his diet to clear liquids and then to a soft diet?

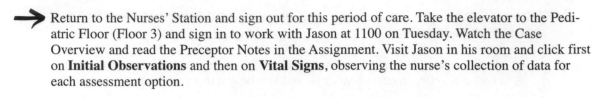 Return to the Nurses' Station and sign out for this period of care. Take the elevator to the Pediatric Floor (Floor 3) and sign in to work with Jason at 1100 on Tuesday. Watch the Case Overview and read the Preceptor Notes in the Assignment. Visit Jason in his room and click first on **Initial Observations** and then on **Vital Signs**, observing the nurse's collection of data for each assessment option.

19. Describe Jason's status on arrival to his room from the PACU in relation to the following issues.

   a. Cardiac and respiratory function:

   b. Orientation and activity:

   c. Pain at operative site:

20. Record Jason's vital signs. Are these readings within normal ranges for an adolescent? Explain.

21. Once Jason is transferred to his room on the Pediatric Floor, he requests that several of his friends be allowed to visit and bring a pizza and movies. In view of his condition, what would be the best response to his request?

22. Adolescents are concerned with their image and how they appear to their friends. How is Jason's current condition likely to affect his self-image? (*Hint:* For information on cognitive and psychosocial development, go to Chapter 16 in your textbook.)

23. Jason may be able to ambulate with crutches on the evening after his surgery. What would be a critical assessment to make before he starts getting out of bed and ambulating?

Diabetes and Musculoskeletal Care

 Reading Assignment: Health Promotion of the Adolescent and Family (Chapter 16)
Pediatric Variations of Nursing Interventions (Chapter 22)
The Child with Endocrine Dysfunction (Chapter 29)
The Child with Musculoskeletal or Articular Dysfunction
(Chapter 31)

Patient: Jason Baker, Room 306

In this lesson the learner will care for an adolescent with type 1 diabetes and a musculoskeletal injury, namely a fractured tibia and fibula, which has been surgically repaired. The learner will examine the effects of the chronic illness on the child and family, as well as the effects that this injury has had on their lifestyle. In this lesson the learner will differentiate the types of insulin and their particular usage in an adolescent undergoing surgery, as well as administration techniques. The learner will also provide care for the adolescent in the postoperative and rehabilitative phase following surgery for a fractured leg, focusing primarily on the musculoskeletal care.

CD-ROM Activity

Go to the Nurses' Station on the Pediatric Floor (Floor 3) and sign in to work with Jason Baker at 1100. After watching the Case Overview and reading the Assignment, open Jason's Chart and review the following sections: History & Physical, Nursing History, Operative Reports, and Progress Notes for Monday and Tuesday. As you review these records, pay close attention to Jason's past history of illnesses and how diabetes has affected (or may yet affect) his present situation.

Writing Activity

1. Jason has had diabetes for about 5 years. Briefly describe the effect of a chronic illness such as diabetes on an adolescent. (*Hint:* To learn more about the impact of illness or disability on the adolescent, refer to Chapter 18 in your textbook.)

2. Define the concept of family-centered care within the context of Jason's family unit. (*Hint:* Family-centered care is introduced in Chapter 1 of your textbook.)

3. Describe the main differences between type 1 diabetes and type 2 diabetes (other than patient's age). (*Hint:* You may want to refer to Chapter 29 in your textbook for assistance.)

4. Identify the three Ps that are the cardinal signs of diabetes. Briefly explain the significance of each term. (*Hint:* Refer to the section on Pathophysiology in Chapter 29 for help.)

5. Identify two long-term complications of diabetes that may directly affect Jason's rehabilitation from the fractured leg. (*Hint:* Refer to Long-Term Complications in Chapter 29.)

6. Because Jason has diabetes, what nursing assessments are carried out in the preoperative and postoperative periods that are especially important in relation to his surgery and fractured leg? (*Hint:* Return to the Operative Reports in Jason's Chart for help.)

Go to Jason's room and observe the nurse perform the assessments you identified in question 6.

7. Below, record your findings from the assessments you just observed in Jason's room.

8. According to the Physician Orders, how often is Jason's blood glucose checked before surgery? What is the significance of periodic blood glucose checks in patients with diabetes who require insulin? What is the role of insulin administration in diabetes?

 Return to Jason's Chart and review the Progress Notes for Tuesday at 0530.

 9. What was Jason's blood glucose level at 0530? What nursing intervention was carried out related to his blood glucose level? How is Jason's surgery likely to affect his diabetes management? (*Hint:* For more information on illness management, refer to Chapter 29 in your textbook.)

10. On the diagram below identify three appropriate sites for insulin administration. Mark each site with an X.

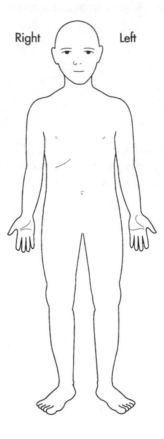

Right   Left

➤ In Jason's Chart, click on **Operative Reports** and review the postoperative orders.

11. What are the postoperative orders for the following in Jason's Chart?

   a. Diet:

   b. Insulin administration:

   c. Frequency of blood glucose checks:

12. What types of insulin preparations are ordered for Jason? What is the rationale for using both types throughout the day?

13. Match each type of insulin with its corresponding characteristics. Each insulin type may have more than one matching characteristic.

_____ Humalog (Lispro H)/ NovoLog (aspart)	a. Rapid-acting insulin
_____ NPH or lente	b. Intermediate-acting insulin
_____ Regular	c. Long-acting insulin
_____ UltraLente	d. Injected immediately before meal
	e. Administered 30 min before meal
	f. Very rapid-acting insulin

14. You have just administered insulin to Jason at 2100 on Tuesday based on a bedside glucose of 275. Fill out the sample MAR below to show the type and amount of insulin you gave him, the method you used to administer it, and the time you gave it. Complete all other necessary information as well.

Patient:	MRN:	Room:	Date:

Medication Administration Record			
Medication	2300–0700	0700–1500	1500–2300

15. Briefly describe how you would draw up the following: Regular insulin 10 units and NPH insulin 50 units. Be specific about the order in which you would complete these steps.

→ Once again, review the History & Physical and Nursing History in Jason's Chart.

16. What do these sections of Jason's Chart reveal about his activity level when he is not ill? How would you counsel Jason to adjust his routine based on his diabetic condition, nutrition, exercise, and right leg injury?

→ Now click on **Operative Reports** and review the postoperative orders again.

17. What orders does Jason have regarding ambulation? Before you ambulate Jason, what would be an important assessment and intervention to minimize complications that may occur since he has been supine and immobile? (*Hint:* Refer to Chapter 31 for more on immobilization and the cardiovascular system.)

18. What are two measures that can be taken to minimize pain in Jason's operated extremity once he returns to bed following ambulation?

19. Later Tuesday evening, Jason ambulates to the bathroom and voids. When he returns to bed, he complains of mild chest pain and dyspnea. He is pale and diaphoretic. What physical assessment criteria should the nurse check (in order of priority) based on Jason's symptoms, diabetic condition, and history of recent surgery?

20. The signs described in question 24 should alert the nurse to a possible

    _____ _____.

 21. List, in order of priority, interventions to establish and maintain Jason's cardiopulmonary and vascular status. (*Hint:* Remember the ABCs. Refer to Chapter 25 in your textbook to learn more about shock and emergency treatment.)

LESSON **21**

Pathophysiology of Asthma

Reading Assignment: The Child with Respiratory Dysfunction (Chapter 23)

Patient: Maria Ortiz, Room 308

The purpose of this lesson is to provide information relating to the factors involved in the etiology of asthma. In particular, the role of allergy will be discussed. The effects of airway inflammation on respiratory symptoms will be discussed, and information will be provided concerning the four levels of asthma severity.

CD-ROM Activity

For this lesson, you will work with Maria Ortiz. Go to the Nurses' Station on the Pediatric Floor (Floor 3) and locate the Login Computer. Sign in to work with Maria at 0700 on Tuesday. After watching the Case Overview and reviewing the Preceptor Note in the Assignment, access Maria's Chart and review her History & Physical.

1. a. List Maria's respiratory signs and symptoms on arrival to the Emergency Department. (*Hint:* Refer to the Pathology of Asthma section in textbook Chapter 32.)

   b. What physiologic component of asthma is responsible for Maria's signs and symptoms in the Emergency Department?

Return to the Nurses' Station and review Maria's Medication Administration Record (MAR).

   2. What medication listed in Maria's MAR is aimed at bringing quick relief from the signs and symptoms that she had in the Emergency Department?

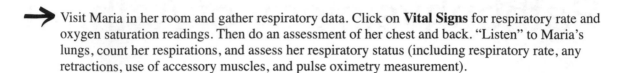 Visit Maria in her room and gather respiratory data. Click on **Vital Signs** for respiratory rate and oxygen saturation readings. Then do an assessment of her chest and back. "Listen" to Maria's lungs, count her respirations, and assess her respiratory status (including respiratory rate, any retractions, use of accessory muscles, and pulse oximetry measurement).

   3. a. Below, list your findings from the room assessment of Maria's respiratory status.

   Respiratory rate:

   Retractions:

   Use of accessory muscles:

   Pulse oximetry measurement:

   b. Now review the section of your textbook on pathophysiology (p. 852). Are Maria's respiratory data consistent with the textbook's description of how increased airway resistance affects the ventilatory status of a child with asthma?

4. Review Box 23-13 (Asthma Severity Classification) on p. 851 of your textbook. Use this information to complete the following table for each of the four classifications of asthma. Then review Maria's History & Physical in her Chart. Place an asterisk next to each description below that applies to Maria.

Classification Criteria	Mild Intermittent	Mild Persistent	Moderate Persistent	Severe Persistent
Daytime Symptoms				
Nighttime Symptoms				
Characteristics of Exacerbations				
Activity Limitations				

5. Based on the information you have recorded in question 4, do you think Maria has mild intermittent, mild persistent, moderate persistent, or severe persistent asthma?

6. Below, list common outdoor and indoor allergens and nonantigenic stimuli that can trigger exacerbations of asthma. Then review Maria's History & Physical in her Chart and place an asterisk next to each allergen or nonantigenic stimulus you found in Maria's Chart that could have triggered her current asthma episode. (*Hint:* If you need help, review Box 23-14 on p. 852 in your textbook.)

Outdoor Allergens	Indoor Allergens	Nonantigenic Stimuli

7. You will need to do some teaching with Maria and her mother about skin tests. Discuss what you would tell them about the specific nursing interventions for a child having skin tests. What can Maria and her mother expect if Maria has skin testing done in the clinic?

8. What types of treatments (not medications) are available to treat the allergic component of asthma? Review Maria's Chart. Has she had any of these treatments? If Maria receives this type of therapy in the future, how would you explain it to her mother?

Signs and Symptoms of Asthma

 Reading Assignment: Physical and Developmental Assessment of the Child
(Chapter 7)
The Child with Respiratory Dysfunction (Chapter 23)

Patient: Maria Ortiz, Room 308

The purpose of this lesson is to provide information relating to the physical assessment of a child with asthma. Specific tests used to diagnose asthma, as well as laboratory and clinical findings will be identified, and the significance of these findings will be discussed.

Writing Activity

Review Physical Assessment of the Chest, Normal and Abnormal Breath Sounds, and Guidelines for Effective Auscultation in Chapter 7 of your textbook, as well as the section on Exacerbation of Asthma in Chapter 32. Write your answers to the following five questions in the table on the next page.

1. Describe the classic signs and symptoms that occur during an asthma exacerbation.

2. List observations the nurse should include in the respiratory assessment of a child with asthma.

3. List the type of breath sound heard over the surface of the lungs, the type heard over the trachea, and the type heard over the bronchi. Identify where the bronchi and trachea bifurcate.

4. List abnormal breath sounds.

5. List auscultation guidelines the nurse should use to effectively hear breath sounds.

1. Classic signs and symptoms of asthma	2. Observations	3. Breath sounds	4. Abnormal breath sounds	5. Auscultation guidelines

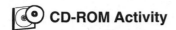 **CD-ROM Activity**

Go to the Nurses' Station on the Pediatric Floor (Floor 3) and sign in to care for Maria Ortiz on Tuesday at 0700. Before you complete the following steps, read questions 6–9 below and keep in mind your answers to questions 1–5.

- Go into Maria's room and watch the nurse perform an assessment of Maria's respiratory system and obtain a set of vital signs.
- Return to the Nurses' Station, open Maria's Chart, and review her Emergency Department Record within the History & Physical section.
- Finally, access Maria's EPR and review the Vital Signs and Respiratory sections.

Questions 6–9 refer to the table of data you created on the previous page. Record your answers directly on that table.

6. Place an asterisk next to any signs, symptoms, or abnormal breath sounds that Maria demonstrated.

7. Place a square beside any findings that were abnormal for Maria. Describe each abnormality.

8. Underline the auscultation guidelines used by Maria's nurse in her respiratory assessment.

9. Circle the physical findings that indicate Maria was having an asthma attack when she came to the ED.

→ Return to Maria's EPR and review her vital signs.

10. Below, record Maria's vital signs data for 0600 on Tuesday. Then list the normal vital signs values for an 8-year-old girl. Are Maria's values within normal limits for her age? If not, circle any vital signs that are abnormal for an 8-year-old child.

Vital Signs	Maria's Vital Signs	Normal Vital Signs for an 8-Year-Old Girl
Temperature		
Heart rate		
Respiratory rate		
Blood pressure		

→ Return to the Nurses' Station and sign out for this period of care. After you have signed out, return to the Login Computer and sign in to work with Maria at 1100. After watching the Case Overview and reading the Preceptor Note within the Assignment, visit Maria's room and assess her respiratory status (including respiratory rate, any retractions, pulse oximetry measurements, adventitious breath sounds, and the presence of cough).

11. Based on your observations of Maria at this time, list any clinical signs and symptoms that indicate a change or worsening of Maria's respiratory condition.

12. Consult your textbook to find what sudden change in breath sounds indicates ventilatory failure and imminent asphyxia in a child with asthma. Based on your findings for question 11, is Maria in danger of ventilatory failure and imminent asphyxia at this time? (*Hint:* If you aren't sure, return to Maria's room and "listen" to her breath sounds again.)

Management and Treatment of Acute Asthma Episodes

 Reading Assignment: Pediatric Variations of Nursing Interventions (Chapter 22)
The Child with Respiratory Dysfunction (Chapter 23)

Patient: Maria Ortiz, Room 308

The purpose of this lesson is to provide information relating to the drugs used to treat acute asthma episodes. The management of status asthmaticus and nursing interventions to be used during an acute asthma episode will also be discussed.

CD-ROM Activity

Go to the Nurses' Station on the Pediatric Floor (Floor 3) and sign in to work with Maria Ortiz at 0700. After watching the Case Overview and reading the Assignment, return to the Nurses' Station. Read questions 1 and 2 below to guide your review of Maria's records and physical assessment. Now open Maria's Chart and review the summary of her admission to the Emergency Department within her History & Physical. Then visit Maria's room and assess her current vital signs, respiratory status, and behavior.

Before answering questions 1 and 2, review Box 23-13 in your textbook.

1. For each assessment area in Column 1 of the table below and on the next page, list your findings for Maria in Column 2, based on your review of Maria's Chart and physical assessment.

Assessment Area	Maria's Data
Talks in	
Alertness	
Respiratory rate	
Accessory muscle use	
Retractions	

Assessment Area	Maria's Data
Wheeze	
Peak expiratory flow rate	
Oxygen saturation	

→ Now access and review Maria's MAR.

2. Is there any evidence that Maria received subcutaneous epinephrine in the Emergency Department or when she got to the Pediatric Unit? Under what circumstances is subcutaneous epinephrine given to a child who is seen in the ED with an acute asthma exacerbation? (*Hint:* You may want to review p. 857 in your textbook.)

→ Return to the Login Computer in the Nurses' Station and sign out for this period of care. Reenter the Login Computer and sign in for Maria at 1300.

3. Which medications were ordered for Maria at the time of admission? Complete the following table with information about these medications. (*Hint:* Return to the Physician Orders in Maria's Chart.)

Name of Medication	Classification or Type of Drug	Rationale for Medication	Dosage, Frequency and Route

→ Return to the Physician's Orders in Maria's Chart to answer question 4.

4. What IV rate was ordered for Maria? Calculate Maria's daily maintenance fluid requirements.

Visit Maria's room and observe the nurse as she assesses Maria's IV site.

    5. What precautions should be taken when infusing IV fluids to a child during an acute asthma episode? Did the nurse include all the necessary observations in her assessment of Maria's IV site? Explain.

 Review Maria's MAR and the Vital Signs and Respiratory Summaries in her EPR as needed to answer question 6.

    6. What is status asthmaticus? Consider the data you reviewed in Maria's EPR and MAR, along with the table you filled out for question 8. Analyze Maria's response to medications, her vital signs, and her respiratory status on admission and throughout the day on Tuesday. Based on the information you have gathered, do you think Maria was ever in status asthmaticus? Give the rationale for your decision.

 Go to Maria's History & Physical and look up her weight.

    7. What is the maximum dose of subcutaneous epinephrine that Maria or any child with asthma should receive during an acute asthma episode?

    8. List several psychosocial nursing interventions that are important for a child having an acute asthma episode. What type of interventions did you see Maria's nurse using? (*Remember:* You may return to Maria's room and replay any of the videos.)

9. How is oxygen given to the child with an asthma exacerbation? How did Maria receive oxygen? Is this consistent with the standards of care for a child with an asthma exacerbation? How much oxygen did Maria receive? Is there any danger in giving too much oxygen to a child with asthma?

10. What nursing interventions are important for a child receiving oxygen? What interventions did you observe Maria's nurse performing?

Patient Education

Reading Assignment: The Child with Respiratory Dysfunction (Chapter 23)

Patient: Maria Ortiz, Room 308

The purpose of this lesson is to identify the two categories of asthma medications and the types of education that the nurse should provide to the child and family about asthma medicines, asthma devices, and health promotion.

CD-ROM Activity

To begin this lesson, go to the Nurses' Station on the Pediatric Floor (Floor 3) and click on the **Login Computer**. Sign in to take care of Maria on Tuesday at 0700. After watching the Case Overview and reading the Assignment, return to the Nurses' Station and open Maria's Chart. Review her History & Physical, Nursing History, and the Physician Orders. Then return to the Nurses' Station and access the MAR. Review Maria's medications prior to coming to the hospital and those prescribed during this hospitalization. The following questions relate to asthma medications in general and to Maria's asthma medications in particular.

1. List the two broad classes of drugs used to treat asthma in your textbook. (*Hint:* Specific information on these drugs can be found on pp. 854–855.)

2. Match each of the following drugs with its correct category. (Note: Drug categories will be used more than once.)

Drug

_____ Cromolyn sodium

_____ Metaproterenol

_____ Nedocromil sodium

_____ Albuterol

_____ Theophylline

_____ Zafirlukast

_____ Budesonide

_____ Solu-medrol

_____ Prelone

Category of Drug

a. Corticosteroid

b. Beta-adrenergic agent

c. Nonsteroidal antiinflammatory

d. Methylxanthine

e. Leukotriene modifier

3. What asthma medication was Maria taking prior to coming to the hospital? How was Maria taking this medication? This medication belongs to which broad class of asthma medications?

4. What is a metered dose inhaler? Was Maria using a metered dose inhaler to take any of her drugs prior to admission?

 5. What is a spacer? When should a child with asthma use a spacer? Did Maria use a spacer to take any of her asthma medications? (_Hint:_ Review pp. 854-855 in your textbook if you need help.)

Now look again at Maria's History & Physical, Nursing History, and Admissions Records in her Chart. As you review these records, think about the areas in which you think Maria and her mother may need additional education or teaching. In particular, think about Maria's presenting signs and symptoms, her food preferences and activities, and their implications for teaching. Make some notes about your thoughts in the space below; then answer the questions on the next page.

Notes

6. List all the steps to be included when teaching Maria how to use her metered dose inhaler effectively.

7. Is there any information in Maria's Chart to indicate that she has used a peak flow meter before this hospitalization? What steps should the nurse include when teaching Maria how to use a peak flow meter when she goes home?

8. Identify the different peak flow meter zones in the following scenario:

Dr. Wools has written an order to be notified if Maria's peak flow rate is less than 90. If 90 is the value that indicates Maria's red peak flow meter zone, what values indicate her yellow and green peak flow meter zones? On the peak flow meter below, draw a straight-line arrow pointing to the beginning value for Maria's yellow peak flow zone and a dotted-line arrow pointing to the value that indicates the beginning of her green peak flow meter zone.

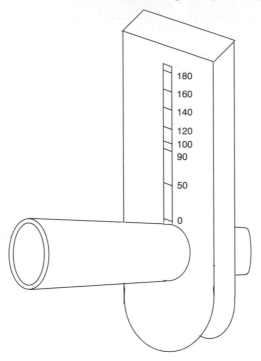

9. What foods may provoke symptoms in some children with asthma? Review Maria's medical records and list any foods Maria enjoys eating that may provoke symptoms.

10. What information about aspirin should the nurse give Maria's mother?

11. List ten things that Maria's mother can do to "allergy-proof" their home. (*Hint:* Refer to p. 855 in your textbook for more information.)

12. a. What should you teach Maria's mother about exercise-induced bronchospasm (EIB) and how to prevent EIB?

b. How can you teach Maria about EIB? Write a brief script for what you would say to Maria to prevent EIB. Use simple, easy-to-understand language.

Discharge Planning and Home Care

👓 **Reading Assignment:** Health Promotion of the School-Age Child and Family
(Chapter 15)
The Child with Respiratory Dysfunction (Chapter 23)

Patient: Maria Ortiz, Room 308

The purpose of this lesson is to discuss aspects of self-management and health promotion for children with asthma and their families and to identify interventions that family members and other individuals can use to foster positive adaptation in the child with asthma.

💿 **CD-ROM Activity**

Go to the Nurses' Station on the Pediatric Floor (Floor 3) and access the Login Computer. Sign in to work with Maria on Tuesday at 1100. Watch the Case Overview and review the Assignment. Then return to the Nurses' Station, open Maria's Chart, and read her History & Physical and Nursing History. After your review, return to the Nurses' Station and read her Kardex. Finally, go into Maria's room and conduct a behavioral assessment. First, click on **Behavior**; then select and observe the videos for the subcategories of Signs of Distress, Needs, Support, and Understanding. Note the interactions in which the nurse asks Maria's mother about her concerns.

1. After reviewing Maria's History of Present Illness when she came to the ED, list specific information about preventing future asthma episodes that you would include in discharge teaching with Maria and her mother.

2. What national and community organizations provide educational programs and brochures that Maria's mother could obtain to help with the self-management of Maria's asthma?

3. Based on your observations of interactions between Maria and her mother and Maria's mother and the nurse, list five interventions that the nurse can use to foster positive adaptation in Maria's family (or in other families that have a child with asthma). Did you observe Maria's nurse using any of these interventions? If so, describe.

→ Once again, enter Maria's room and observe the assessment video that deals with Behavior. Observe the interactions between Maria and the nurse, this time paying close attention to the interactions under the subcategory of Activity.

4. What interventions does the nurse use to help Maria cope with the anxiety of hospitalization? What activities does the nurse suggest for Maria? Are these activities age-appropriate for Maria?

5. a. What grade is Maria in at school? If you were the nurse at Maria's school, what information about a child with asthma would you want to receive?

   b. What specific information would you want to receive from Maria's mother?

6. The school coach has been concerned about Maria and has done some research about asthma. The coach asks you whether there are any play activities that elementary school children with asthma can do to improve their expiratory breathing time. What activities would you recommend to the coach?

7. Maria's science teacher asks you whether any substances or animals in the school classroom could trigger an asthma episode in Maria or any other child with asthma. What guidance would you give the science teacher?

8. What is an Asthma Action Plan? Return to Maria's Chart and read the Nursing Admissions Pediatric Patient Profile in the Nursing History. List any information that would have been included on Maria's preadmission Asthma Action section.

→ Within Maria's Chart, review her current Physician Orders and History & Physical. Then return to the Nurses' Station and access her MAR. Review these records as needed to answer the following questions.

9. Has she ever had theophylline prescribed for her asthma? If Dr. Wools decides to prescribe theophylline for treatment of Maria's nighttime asthma symptoms when she is discharged, what is the maximum serum level of this drug recommended for outpatient care?

10. What should you teach Maria's mother about the early signs of theophylline toxicity?